THE Fasting *Bible*

HOW TO LOSE WEIGHT, GROW YOUNGER AND HEAL YOUR BODY (IN 30 DAYS OR LESS)

*By **Lynn Hardy**, **ND**, **CNC***

Disclaimer

The information presented is the author's opinion and does not constitute any health or medical advice. The content of this book is for informational purposes only and is not intended to diagnose, treat, cure, or prevent any condition or disease.

Please seek advice from your healthcare provider for your personal health concerns prior to taking healthcare advice from this book.

Table of Contents

My Fasting Story

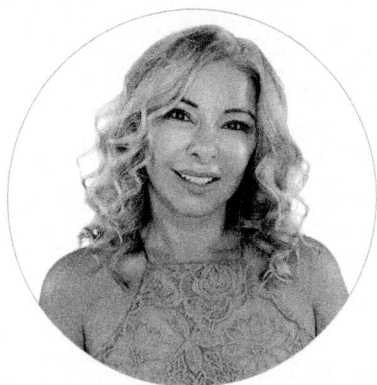

JUICE FASTING WAS QUITE POPULAR IN THE 90S AND I WAS HAPPY TO jump on that bandwagon, especially because it promised rapid weight loss. This means I started fasting in my early 20s. I would fast drinking nothing but fruit and vegetable juices throughout the day for 2-3 weeks at a time a couple of times a year. I was also organizing community juice fasts where we would fast together as a group, and it was very powerful and motivating for everyone.

I have tried every type of fast out there throughout the years, and I can honestly say that fasting is still part of my regular health routine.

The fast that had the biggest impact on my life was a 10-day water fast 5 years ago.

I just took it day by day, it was the first time I was water fasting and I certainly didn't set out to do such an extended fast., Yet, I carried on as I was feeling amazing and my body was going through the most incredible transformation.

This was the fast that really started my weight loss; I ended up losing 25 lbs.

This was not an easy task being perimenopausal. But that's not all, I was also able to heal a 2-year shoulder injury and I got rid of my eczema once and for all. What's more, it helped tremendously with my Hashimoto's thyroiditis, and I felt like my metabolism was finally reset and my health restored. I was hooked!

Therefore, since then, I've completed several water fasts, I do intermittent fasting every day, and I've even completed several dry fasts. I'm now 52 and feel healthier and stronger than I was in my 20s. I also weigh the same and fit into the same clothes as when I was 25.

I truly believe that we are designed to feast and fast and that this is the best way to achieve the optimal health, energy, and vitality we all dream of.

Fasting has become very popular again in recent years and it seems like a new way to fast pops up each day. I see a lot of people who wish to fast but they're simply confused by all the different and sometimes conflicting information out there. This is why I decided to write *The Fasting Bible*. I want to help people not only to make sense of all the different methods, but also find the right fast for their needs and lifestyle.

Fasting shouldn't be difficult or confusing.

I sincerely hope this book will help guide you into the wonderful world of fasting and I can't wait to hear your success story. You can find me on social media and YouTube under *The Aging Games*. Speaking of which, my YouTube channel is another hub of important information; there you will find detailed videos about the different fasts and much more.

Plus, I love reading you, so please don't hesitate to reach out to me with a message at any time.

Love,
Lynn

CHAPTER 1

The History of Fasting

FASTING IS AS OLD AS MANKIND. STORIES ABOUT FASTING DECORATE history with ancient tales of healings, spiritual miracles, and even beliefs of immortality through the practice. Today there has been a resurgence in fasting practices as many people are recognizing the health and healing benefits it can provide. Some even claim that fasting is not a fad, but a cure–if done correctly, of course.

One of the earliest and most recognizable stories of fasting dates back to biblical times when Jesus is said to have left his community to spend 40 days fasting in the desert. During this time, it is said that angels ministered to him while Satan tempted him. And thanks to what is claimed to be renewed strength gained from the fast, not only did he survive, but Jesus went on to a service of public ministry, performed miracles, and even defeated death.

Today members of Catholicism fast when observing Lent, as they reflect to acknowledge a period of darkness that precedes light, while members of the Church of Latter-Day Saints are encouraged to fast by abstaining from both food and water for a full 24 hours at least once each month. Muslims are also instructed to fast during

Ramadan to remind them of others who have suffered before them. Moreover, this fasting also brings them closer to Allah, or God. Some religious leaders call church members to fast as a symbolic gesture to bring awareness to and raise money for victims of disasters, while other religious leaders have fasted in the name of protest.

It is clear that some cultures believe fasting rewards the practitioner with a clear mind ready to accept visions, or an open mind with direct access to the spiritual world. Fasting was also equated with purifying the body and mind, thus allowing one to become more "divine," or closer to God. Overall, the practice of fasting seems to be an elixir for the body and mind for both spiritual practitioners and spiritual healers. The religious history of fasting provides some insight into the idea that fasting not only improves mental acuity, but seems to have a brain-boosting benefit that helps awaken the senses, even those we are unaware of.

Current research shows that fasting improves alertness, cognitive function, and memory all while allowing the body's inherent healing abilities to awaken. In addition, fasting seems to lead to an increase in both emotional and physical well-being.[1] In fact, some laboratory studies show that fasting stimulates the production of a nerve protein that is critical in the generation of nerve cells

---

1   Wilhelmi de Toledo F, Grundler F, Bergouignan A, Drinda S, Michalsen A. Safety, health improvement and well-being during a 4 to 21-day fasting period in an observational study including 1422 subjects. PLoS One. 2019;14(1):e0209353. Published 2019 Jan 2. doi:10.1371/journal.pone.0209353

of the hippocampus; an area of the brain that is related to emotional regulation, especially in the recalling of positive memories.[2] No wonder many people who fast feel renewed!

Fasting for Physical Healing

Aside from religious fasting, abstaining from food in the natural world is also common practice. When animals are sick or injured, their first reaction or instinct is to stop eating. This is true in all animals including mice and dogs. This may be because digestion consumes a high amount of physical energy, so abstaining from food may allow the body to direct energies into regeneration and healing. At the same time, many holistic practitioners believe that healing begins in the gut, and allowing this system to rest allows it, and every organ connected to it, to rest and reset.

Digestion requires great amounts of energy and some health professionals claim that when too much energy is directed to digestion, there will be less energy for physical energy and brain power. Overeating, which is the opposite of fasting, takes an even larger toll on digestion and can leave you feeling fatigued and sometimes physically ill. But there are other reasons why a person might feel awful after a meal.

> **FAST FACT**
>
> Fasting relieves the gut of leftover food and fecal remnants and allows it to regenerate. This automatically has a positive impact on our immune system, since around 70 percent of all of the body's immune cells are located in the gut.

2   Anand KS, Dhikav V. Hippocampus in health and disease: An overview. Ann Indian Acad Neurol. 2012;15(4):239-246. doi:10.4103/0972-2327.104323

FAST FACT

During hunter-gatherer days, the hunters were in a fasted state while searching for food.

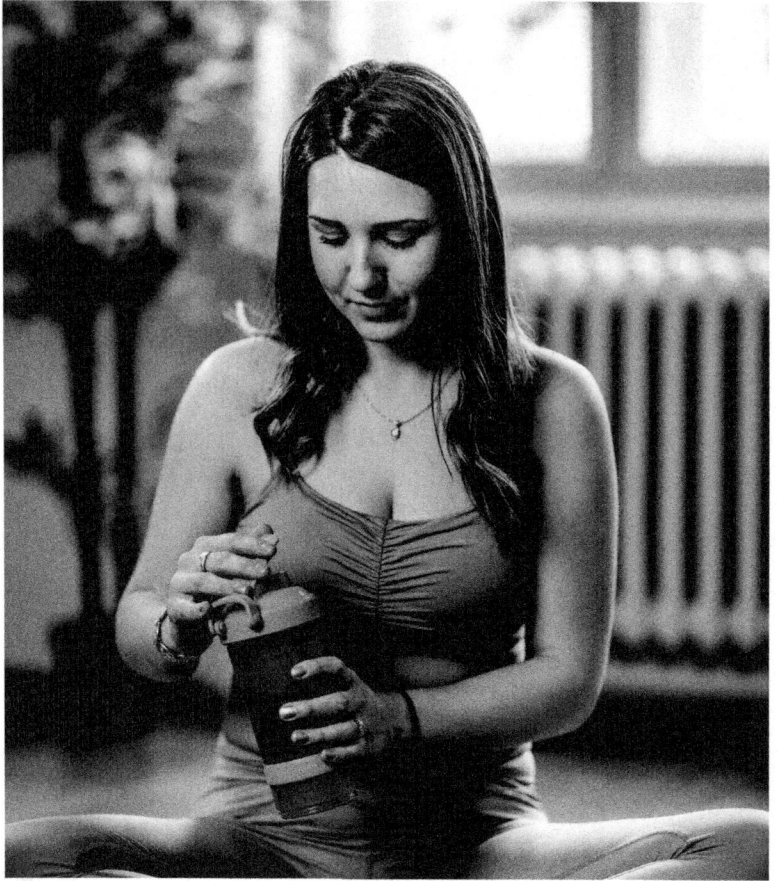

Today's food is an industry with products that are laden with chemical additives to enhance the flavor, color, and shelf life of foods. Some foods contain animal hormones that may not mix well with ours. Furthermore, food processing strips nutrients while adding chemicals and fake vitamins that are often not digestible. And lastly, genetically modified foods are not always what they seem. For example, fish genes may be added to strawberries (unfortunate for those who enjoy fruit, but are allergic to fish) and pesticides are grown right into corn, which cannot be washed away. Altogether, these alterations can wreak havoc on our digestion. No wonder fasting is becoming popular again!

Fasting allows your body and digestion to take a rest. When rested, your body kicks in to promote a process called autophagy, in which the cells dissolve and remove damaged and worn-out cells or portions of cells, and another process called autolysis, in which the body breaks down diseased tissues and even tumor-like growths. And this is only the beginning of the benefits that fasting has to offer.

Many people enjoy more energy while fasting and immediately feel lighter and more clear-headed. Of course, not everyone feels the same, because your body will react according to your level of health and the processes it must go through on the path to healing. Fasting is a tool that can be used to promote these miraculous processes.

Unfortunately, we are too often instructed to eat in an attempt to add nutrients to help the body heal. Some people may still follow the old tradition of "feed a cold, starve a fever," and so abstain from food during certain illnesses. But if we can get over this mindset, many people might find that it is possible to heal without food, and in fact, we may be built to fast.

The Myths of Fasting

Fasting has gotten a bad rap in the last century due to myths from misguided health and medical professionals. Contrary to popular belief, fasting will not cause starvation and will not slow your metabolism. The following are some of the common myths of fasting and how they have been debunked.

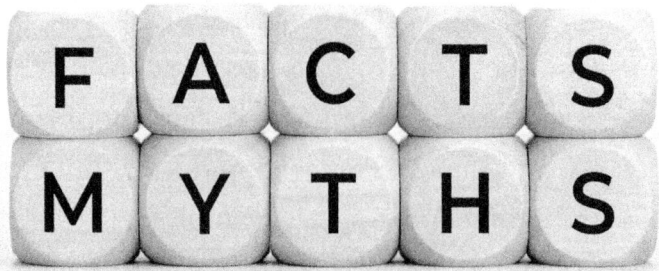

- **Myth: Fasting slows your metabolism.** This is false, as studies show that intermittent fasting, or fasting alternated with normal caloric intake results in weight loss and improved metabolism, compared to calorie-restrictive diets.[3] However, calorie restriction alone results in a much slower metabolism as well as muscle loss. In fact, it is common for dieters who follow calorie restrictive dieting alone to gain back the weight they lost.

- **Myth: Fasting makes you weak.** This is true for those embarking on very long fasts. But normal or average fasting of a few days as well as intermittent fasting results in increased energy for most people, which is why it is one of the most popular health practices today.

- **Myth: Fasting causes binge eating.** This is also not true for the average person. Those with eating disorders may be triggered; however, eating disorders are contraindicated within fasting programs. For most people, fasting helps control appetite and

---

3   Leonie K Heilbronn, Steven R Smith, Corby K Martin, Stephen D Anton, Eric Ravussin, Alternate-day fasting in nonobese subjects: effects on body weight, body composition, and energy metabolism, The American Journal of Clinical Nutrition, Volume 81, Issue 1, January 2005, Pages 69–73, https://doi.org/10.1093/ajcn/81.1.69

improve the functions of hormones, including ghrelin, the hunger hormone.

- **Myth: Fasting reduces brain power.** Again, this is false as during fasting, the body begins to use ketones for energy, which is a superior form of energy for brain cells. In addition, fasting promotes the ancient instinct of survival, which was a necessary state that allowed our ancestors to stay alert and alive until the next hunt.

Hunting, Gathering and Fasting

Our human ancestors hunted for food and, when they were successful, often had entire communities to feed. Before farming, humans could easily starve before they were successful at finding their next meal. Depending on the location and climate, there may have been fruits, roots, mushrooms and other things they could gather between hunts–but these would provide very few calories for sustenance.

Nevertheless, they still had the physical energy and mental acuity to continue in search of the next hunt for protein and stay safe from predators at the same time. It is likely then that the human body has an internal mechanism that allows for feasting and fasting, and this would explain why people feel more energetic and mentally alert while fasting. Moreover, it would also explain why humans are lethargic after a large meal, instead of full of energy thanks to the so many calories (which are supposedly energy) flowing through the digestive tract.

It seems the many fasting plans of today actually mimic the feast or famine instinct with protocols that promote fasting two out of every seven days. Other similar plans call for eating only one meal a day, while still others claim the most effective fast is to not eat for 16 hours a day with an 8-hour "feeding window." Each of these is a form of intermittent fasting, or allowing yourself to feast and then giving digestion a rest.

Extended Fasting

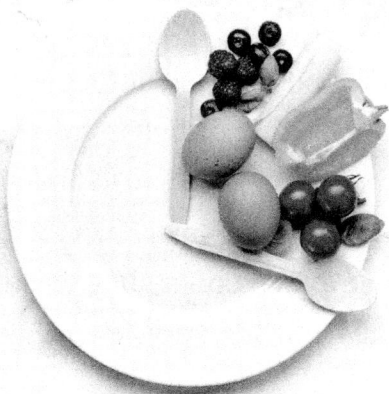

One controversial subject is a person's proclivity for what was once known as religious fasting, holy anorexia, or "anorexia mirabilis," which translates as "miraculous lack of appetite." St. Catherine of Siena, a patron saint of Italy, was considered a mystic and a political activist, and was regarded for her spiritual visions. And she was well known for her extended fasting practices, which the church claimed was evidence of saintliness.

However, Catherine wasn't the only female known for her holy anorexia. Religious women of medieval times abstained from food to show their devotion to God and to demonstrate their strength of inner spirit. Giri Bala was an Indian saint who was said to not have eaten in over 50 years, and when visited by the famous Paramahansa Yogananda, was still of healthy weight and had healthy, toned skin. When asked how she survived, she claimed it was due to energies of the air, sunshine, and cosmic power that recharged the body.

These stories are certainly not to advocate fasting for months or years at a time. While we know that today many women are prone to anorexia, it seems to be for the wrong reasons, which is why they get sick due to improper use of fasting. The point is, what is this seemingly inherent instinct to abstain from food for a set length of time? Maybe the answer was discovered as far back as the beginnings of Western Medicine.

"Fasting is the Greatest Remedy, the Physician Within"

The above quote is credited to a great healer named Paracelsus, who was one of the first physicians who combined chemistry with medicine. He was against the ancient practice of bloodletting and believed in healing therapies that did not disturb the body. Even though the mainstream thought during his time in the 1500s was to drain blood so that the circulatory system could purify itself, Paracelsus believed fasting was the answer and promoted it as a way to help the body heal itself.

Before Paracelsus was Hippocrates (460-357BC), who is commonly known today as the father of modern medicine. He also promoted the idea that the body is self-healing and was an advocate of fasting. In fact, he promoted water fasting for most illnesses or diseases even in the acute stage. Even Plato was an advocate of fasting as he claimed that he did so for greater physical health as well as mental acuity. Included in this elite class are Aristotle, Galen, and Avicenna, who are all documented as recommending fasts as a healing tool for their patients.

In Greek medicine, it is believed that we thrive on something called "Innate Heat," which is akin to an internal, metabolic fire that is constantly burning. Fire requires fuel and, when we eat, the nutrients are the fuel that is burned. But when we abstain from eating, the metabolic fire requires another supply of fuel, and so it feeds on internal reserves and begins by "cleaning house." This is the act that is referred to in Greek literature as the Inner Physician. During this time, the body digests excess wastes and toxins, or what modern researchers are just now discovering as the processes of autophagy and autolysis.

Spiritual masters from nearly every culture require their students to cleanse and purify their bodies and minds by fasting before they begin training. Fasting helps one to overcome food addictions so the mind can focus on spiritual matters. According to biologists, a natural ancestral instinct is to be extremely aware during fasting so that the mind and body are ready for the next hunt. It seems our ancestors also found a way to exploit this trait for spiritual purposes.

"Everyone has a physician inside him or her; we just have to help it in its work. The natural healing force within each one of us is the greatest force in getting well. Our food should be our medicine. Our medicine should be our food. But to eat when you are sick is to feed your sickness."– Hippocrates

---

Lessons from Ancient Medicine

Today we are learning that many practices attributed to folklore had at least some validity all along. We know the health benefits of chicken soup go beyond just making you warm. It turns out the broth is rich in proteins and fatty acids that promote cell repair throughout your entire body. Bloodletting led to the current medical specialty known as phlebotomy, and the use of the herb willow bark for pain is the basis for the current medicine that we call aspirin. Healing practices from our history continue to be the foundation for much of the modern medicinal practices still in use today.

While we do have many stories about fasting used in ancient medicine, the true origin of the practice is unknown. Some anthropologists speculate it is because we are part of the animal kingdom and fasting is simply an inherent survival instinct. When sick or hurt, it is natural to not have an appetite and the fasting instinct may be a function that allows the body to heal itself.

According to Leonard Guarente, the Novartic Professor of Biology at the Glenn Laboratory for the Science of Aging at MIT, fasting is a prehistoric survival adaptation so that humans could survive "between hunts." During fasting, he noted, certain central bodily systems slow down, women become less fertile and even the aging process slows down.

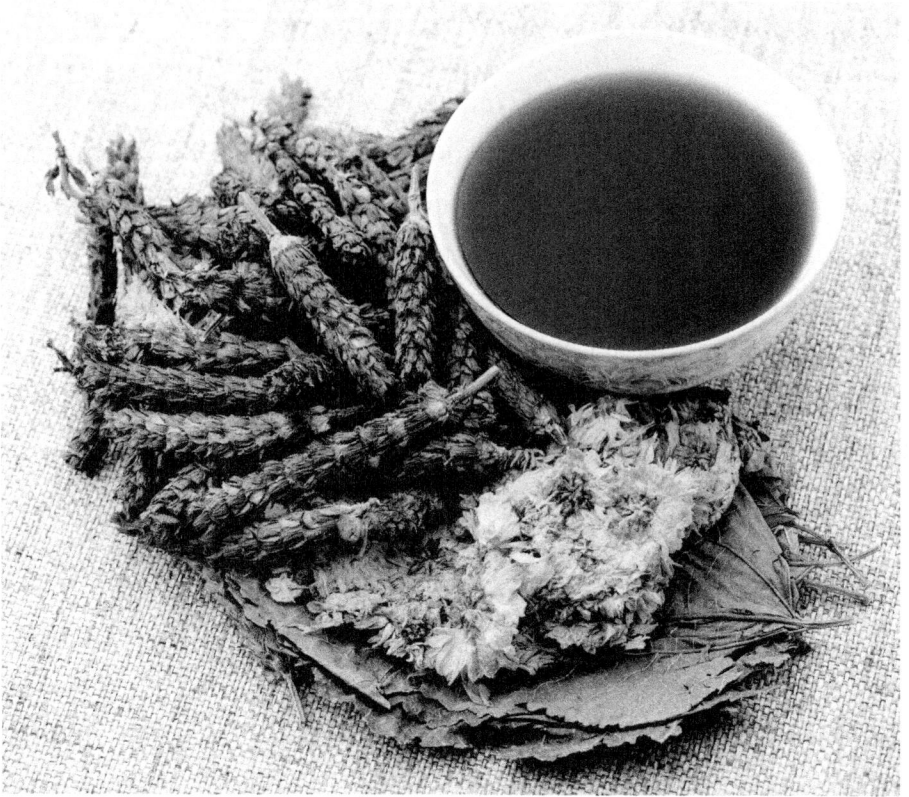

Today we have proof that fasting helps the body heal. New research has shown the benefits of fasting to help fight chronic disease as it reduces chronic internal inflammation, which is a hindrance to healing. And better yet, fasting does not interfere with your body's immune response to acute infections like most foods do.[4]

Recent research is showing that extended or prolonged fasting stimulates the immune system. In one study, fasting for 48 to 120 hours enhanced the body's ability to fight toxins and stress, and increased

---

4   Michalsen A, Li C. Fasting therapy for treating and preventing disease–current state of evidence. Forsch Komplementmed. 2013;20(6):444-53. doi: 10.1159/000357765. Epub 2013 Dec 16. PMID: 24434759.

cell protection. Fasting also promoted stem cell renewal, which is another important factor in self-healing.[5]

More evidence about fasting stimulating the body's ability to heal lies in other studies. One peer-reviewed study from 2015 found that both fasting and keto diets reduced internal inflammation, a factor in many chronic diseases while promoting the use of fatty acids for energy.[6]

The implications of the above studies are that fasting promotes a healing response in multiple body systems and through various mechanisms and channels. It seems to stimulate an improved immune response, help the body regenerate healthy immune cells, and trigger internal cell healing mechanisms. On the other hand, intermittent fasting may be just as effective as a keto diet to lose excess body fat. Next, we will explore fasting in the modern world.

> **FAST FACT**
>
> When we fast, the body does not have its usual access to glucose, forcing the cells to resort to other means and materials to produce energy.

5   Cheng CW, Adams GB, Perin L, et al. Prolonged fasting reduces IGF-1/PKA to promote hematopoietic-stem-cell-based regeneration and reverse immunosuppression [published correction appears in Cell Stem Cell. 2016 Feb 4;18(2):291-2]. Cell Stem Cell. 2014;14(6):810-823. doi:10.1016/j.stem.2014.04.014

6   Youm YH, Nguyen KY, Grant RW, et al. The ketone metabolite β-hydroxybutyrate blocks NLRP3 inflammasome-mediated inflammatory disease. Nat Med. 2015;21(3):263-269. doi:10.1038/nm.3804

CHAPTER 2

Fasting in the Modern World

NOW THAT WE KNOW FASTING IS AS OLD AS MANKIND AND PROBA-
bly encoded within our genes, why is it then that we are seeing a resurgence in fasting practices? Sadly, there are many valid
reasons, beginning with the fact that in spite of the so-called ad-
vances in modern medicine, people are fatter and sicker than ever
before in history. As far as the Hippocratic oath, "Do No Harm,"
over 200,000 people die every year as a direct result of medical
treatment, with some estimates being even higher because less than
10% of medical errors are reported.[7] In Europe, the only mea-
surement of these reports is from the British Journal of Medicine,
which calculated in 2016 an annual average of 251,000 deaths
from medical errors.[8]

---

7   Anderson JG, Abrahamson K. Your Health Care May Kill You: Medical Errors. Stud Health Technol Inform. 2017;234:13-17. PMID: 28186008.

8   Makary M A, Daniel M. Medical error—the third leading cause of death in the US BMJ 2016; 353 :i2139 doi:10.1136/bmj.i2139

With the overall population becoming sicker and taking medications, an awakening is also taking place. People are learning to take control of their health and are seeing that health is not necessarily about taking pharmaceuticals. We have the ability to take charge of our own health and put off chronic disease and a lifetime of medications, or avoid them altogether.

Even as people are becoming more health conscious in an effort to avoid illness, modern life has taken its toll. Schedules have become overly busy, thus making fast food or quick meals a necessity for many. We have been trained that starving is unhealthy and that missing meals will slow our metabolism, thus causing weight gain. As you will soon learn, this is not true.

For those who are trying their hardest to get fit and healthy, more and more fake health foods are populating the market shelves. We are consuming protein bars, fake meats, canned vegetables, and dried fruits in the name of health. Unfortunately, labeling and advertising laws allow companies to deceive consumers into believing that certain foods are healthy when they are harmful. Contributing to these practices are the unhealthy government dietary guidelines that instruct people to overeat starchy foods while avoiding fats and other nutrients the body needs for healthy functioning.

Government Dietary Guidelines

Government dietary guidelines are supposed to serve the general public at large and help in preventing disease. One of the issues, however, is there is no differentiation between healthy and unhealthy foods. In the eyes of the "food pyramid" of America, the

UK "Eatwell Plate," or the Spanish Wheel, grains are grains, meats are meats, and fats are just fats. But this is extremely misleading.

For example, grains are one of the largest contributors to digestive problems. Instead of true whole grains that contain protein, healthy fats, and fiber, most "grain" foods are made with a ghostlike version of whole grains, often called whole wheat. These foods are often touted as healthy, but in most cases, the bran, germ, and endosperm of the grains are separated and altered. This way, only the remnants of the grains, which have very few nutrients (if any at all) are left. These are called refined grains.

Refined grains contain only the endosperm which is then dried, bleached, and pulverized into a powder. The powder is used to make breads, cereals, pastas, crackers, tortillas, and any other foods that are wheat based. Many "whole grain" foods also use the same powder, but manufacturers then add whole oats, seeds and nuts, so they can claim the whole grain label. Added to this are synthetic vitamins like niacin and riboflavin along with sugar, colorings, and preservatives to give the food a nice, long shelf life and a hint of nutrition, which they market as "fortified" and healthy.

According to cardiologist William Davis, MD, author of the book *Wheat Belly*, modern wheat is also a product of genetic engineering and turns out to be a hindrance not

> **FAST FACT**
>
> Studies of fasting rats show improvement in both brain structure and growth of nerve cells that improve brain function.

only to digestion but can lead to skin problems like eczema, weight gain, emotional issues, and heart disease. It is true that grains today have synthesized components that were not in ancient grains. No wonder so many people are ridden with ill health today!

However, genetically altered grains are not our only worries. Unbeknownst to many, food engineering has been used for decades to intentionally stimulate cravings. Scientists are employed by food manufacturers to learn how much sugar is needed to create the "bliss point" of sweetness that keeps you expecting more. This technology is then used in breads, cereals, and even salad dressings. Science and data are used to learn what makes humans attracted to food and know full well that sugar stimulates hormones like dopamine much in the same way as cocaine. Food addiction is not a problem of those with an "addictive" disposition, but something that is engineered in the name of corporate profits.

Misguided Diet Advice

Along with the misinformation about our foods, many people are misinformed about healthy eating practices. For example, one claim is that we need to constantly consume nutrition to keep blood sugar levels healthy, especially if you are diabetic or pre-diabetic. However, snacking may be a culprit that hinders the path to health. This is because the time between meals is when your insulin levels naturally decrease, which then allows stored sugars in fat cells and the liver, known as glycogen, to be used for energy. But when we are constantly snacking, this function never takes place, resulting in more and more sugar being stored in fat cells, as they increase in size.

Other misinformation was in the zero-fat craze, which began in America in the 1950s. During this time, many people were living lavish lifestyles with rich foods like steak in lobster sauce or buttery vegetables with rich breads and potatoes that were consumed together in overly indulgent meals. This was the era when the first set of dietary guidelines came about, which advocated for consuming a very low-fat diet, and to replace fatty dairy and meats with carbohydrates like bread and pasta. And then came the rise of obesity and adverse health epidemics including digestive issues, as we saw above.

Since the 1950s there have been thousands of diet and nutritional plans and gimmicks. Some call for measuring portions, counting calories, and breaking down the macronutrients in all your foods. There are even apps to help you monitor your micronutrients and count how many calories you burn. It sounds like one must be a scientist simply to be healthy! This, I believe, is why fasting is not only becoming more popular, but is an important health tool that is needed more than ever before.

How Fasting Became Popular, Again

Fasting is one of the easiest ways to reset your metabolism and begin the path to regaining your health. Water fasting is the easiest form of fasting, but because of the atrocities that have taken place in our food supply by the food industry, not everyone is healthy enough to jump into this practice. Besides, some preparations are necessary, but more on that later.

The popularity of fasting is rising because of the vast number of people with health and weight problems, and because of the confusion about what diet plan is the best to follow. I believe deep down our instincts are telling us that we need to get back to the simplicity of fasting to allow the inner physician to begin its healing processes. Aside from preparing for a fast, it requires no calorie counting or measurements of macronutrient ratios in relation to daily calories, individual weights and goals. The simplicity makes it not only doable but achievable.

Fasting addresses the insulin problem (often caused by snacking) by allowing insulin levels to go down long enough to burn fat as we are meant to. It can help reset digestion, improve metabolism, stabilize blood sugar, and promote cellular cleansing resulting in lowering our risk for cancers and other chronic diseases. It can lessen internal, chronic inflammation thus reducing pain and enhancing brain function.

Embarking on a fast requires no money for gimmicks like specialized drinks, supplements or exercise equipment. Water fasting requires no juice making while techniques, like intermittent fasting (IF), do not require a special diet. This is particularly appealing for those who want to lose weight and for those who want to turn back time, since calorie restriction is known to promote longevity.

We can say, then, that fasting is effective thanks to the fact that it is as old as mankind and to science proving how it can help improve fitness, protect from obesity, reduce the risk of metabolic diseases, and it can even be successfully used as a weight loss tool.

According to a scientific review of data collected from the World Health Organization, Medline, PubMed and others, about one in three people suffer from multiple chronic diseases, globally.[9] Luckily, some leaders from the Institute for Functional Medicine are showing how fasting improves fatty liver, insulin resistance, and has even helped some patients reverse type 2 diabetes, making them no longer need insulin.

Today, many people are becoming more aware that as they age, they may not want to be beholden to their health insurance or pharmaceuticals to keep them alive. Growing old gracefully and healthily is everyone's right and can be achieved through calorie restriction and fasting, as proven by more than a few animal studies.

Fasting and the Passionate Promoters

There are many professionals that have researched and found fasting to be an effective way to improve health. Promoters of fasting range from medical doctors to holistic professionals and everyday people who have greatly benefitted from the practice and want to share their stories and inspire anyone who will listen. The following are some of the outstanding people who have contributed to bringing fasting back into the spotlight.

Dr Otto Buchinger was a German physician who specialized in internal medicine. He discovered fasting when he became incapable of working due to severe joint rheumatism. He is credited with the first systematic study of fasting and its positive effect on vari-

9   Hajat C, Stein E. The global burden of multiple chronic conditions: A narrative review. Prev Med Rep. 2018;12:284-293. Published 2018 Oct 19. doi:10.1016/j.pmedr.2018.10.008

ous diseases. He stated that, "During fasting, the body thrives, but the soul hungers," to which he countered that one who is fasting should be provided with spiritual food, which he coined, "dietetics for the soul."

Dr. Jason Fung is a Canadian-based nephrologist (kidney doctor) that brought attention to the science behind intermittent fasting and how it successfully helps people lose weight. In his book, *The Obesity Code*, he lays out the science of fasting and low-carb eating and how these help people lose weight. After noticing that simply restricting calories helps people lose weight, the science backed up what he suspected: that simply lowering calories will result in a slower metabolism and eventually regaining the weight. But intermittent fasting works with the body's natural circadian rhythm, ceasing the constant insulin elevations while allowing time for the digestion and hormonal system to rest and reset, thus making it easier to keep the weight off.

Jimmy Moore is an author and blogger who has written several books on nutrition. Even though his degree is in political science and public policy, he became well known for his journey from a dangerous weight of 410 lbs (185 kg). Interestingly, he co-authored a book with Dr. Fung called *The Complete Guide to Fasting* and also teamed up with nutritional researcher Dr. Eric Westman, to write *Cholesterol Clarity*, where they analyze newer perspectives on healthy cholesterol levels.

Dr. Mindy Pelz is the owner of Family Life Wellness and enjoys the nickname of "The Reset Doc." She guides her fans through fasting and detoxing heavy metals. Her passion stems from a past diagnosis of Chronic Fatigue Syndrome (CFS) related to the Epstein-Barr virus. She suffered from brain fog, extreme fatigue, and muscle wasting until she discovered how to take charge of her health. Fasting is one of her core tools for health and energy.

Dr. Yeral Patel is a functional medicine physician in Newport Beach, CA who specializes in anti-aging and regenerative medicine. Intermittent fasting is included in her protocols to help improve mental clarity, increase energy, improve metabolism and insulin levels, and slow the aging process. In her practice, she advocates fasting a full one to two days each week as a safe way to maintain or improve overall health.

Gin Stephens is the author of the book, *Fast. Feast. Repeat.*, in which she discusses various ways to incorporate intermittent fasting into your lifestyle. Her advocacy stems from a successful 80-pound weight loss thanks to IF, and she now hosts a podcast where she interviews doctors and others who promote fasting as a way of life.

Maria Emmerich has helped millions of people lose weight and get healthy through her delicious keto recipes and Protein Sparing Modified Fasts (PSMF). Having lost 80 pounds herself and reversed her PCOS and IBS, Maria started writing books about the Keto lifestyle 20 years ago. She is Halle Berry's favorite author and has done cooking videos with Halle on her Instagram.

David Asprey is the author of the book *Fast This Way: Burn Fat, Heal Inflammation, and Eat Like the High-Performing Human You Were Meant to Be*. A pioneer of the Biohacking movement, Dave has devoted his life to elevating human performance using the latest scientific research combined with ancient healing traditions, including fasting.

Krista Varady, PhD, is a Professor of Nutrition at the University of Illinois – Chicago. She has received numerous grants from prestigious groups like the National Institutes of Health, International Life Sciences Institute, and the American Heart Association for her research involving IF for weight loss and maintenance as well as heart health for obese patients.

Dr. Eric Berg is a chiropractor and health educator who practiced in Virginia in the United States for nearly 30 years. He advocates IF as a way to lose weight, reset metabolism, and increase growth hormone, which is key to anti-aging.

Dr. Michael Mosley is a former doctor who was named Medical Journalist of the Year by the British Medical Association and has written numerous books on fasting. He made famous the 5:2 diet, which advocates a form of IF in which you eat "normal" for five days and greatly restrict calories to around 500 per day for two days each week. While his program is criticized by some because of the lack of healthy food requirements, some find it an easy approach to begin controlling the appetite.

Dr. Sergey Filonov is the world's foremost authority on the most extreme form of fasting: dry fasting. As the author of several books on the topic, Dr. Filonov also hosts 10-day dry fasting retreats in Montenegro.

Fasting has been used in Europe as a medical treatment for years. Often called fasting therapy, there are literally hundreds, if not thousands, of spas and treatment centers where one can go for a fasting vacation. Tens of thousands of people use these retreats every year to help their bodies reset and heal while medical personnel keep track of blood pressure and oversee blood tests.

According to Dr. Sandrine Thuret, a French researcher at King's College in London, intermittent fasting is one of the quickest ways to improve memory and promote neurogenesis, which is the ability of the body to generate new neurons or brain cells. She believes the positive benefits to the brain are threefold; fewer toxins in the cerebral spinal fluid of the brain, an increase in neurons, and the presence of ketone bodies, which is a highly efficient form of fuel for the brain.

The prestigious Karger Journal, based in Basel, Switzerland is a peer-reviewed journal that publishes scientific and medical journals from many disciplines, including cellular physiology and biochemistry, kidney and blood pressure research, and cardiology. In 2013, the review article entitled *Fasting Therapy – an Expert Panel of Update of the 2002 Consensus Guidelines* stated that fasting therapy is an established therapeutic medical approach within specialized hospitals and clinical departments for integrative medicine.

The review goes on to explain how fasting has been beneficial for many chronic diseases, as well as metabolic diseases, chronic inflammatory conditions, and even psychosomatic disorders. Fasting also benefits healthy people, as it may be applied to the prevention of disease, according to the review's authors.

Fasting has gained popularity in American alternative medicine over the past several decades, and many doctors feel it is beneficial. The latest research is showing that health practitioners who have always promoted cleansing and fasting were right; the health benefits are numerous and fasting provides a time during which the human body heals itself.

At the same time, some prominent medical doctors advocate fasting in their practices to help their patients heal. Angela Fitch, MD and associate director at the Massachusetts General Hospital Weight Center has used IF with her patients to help them lose weight. LF Amaral, a Research and Clinical Registered Dietician at Cedars-Sinai Samuel Oschin Cancer Center supports IF as an option with some of her cancer patients. This trend seems to be growing as researchers learn more and doctors see improved results.

Fasting is a central therapy in detoxification, a healing method founded on the principle that the buildup of toxic substances in the body is responsible for many illnesses and conditions. What was once considered a New Age fantasy is now a proven fact; fasting stimulates a process called au-tophagy, which is the ability of the body to destroy and remove damaged cells, allowing the body to regenerate new, healthy cells. This benefit, in addition to the other known benefits that fasting is widely used for, such as stabilizing blood sugar, resetting digestion, and reigning in appetite, point to what the early leaders of health and healing have always known: that fasting is a powerful tool and maybe even central to a healthy life.

CHAPTER 3

Different Types
of Fasting

JUST AS THERE ARE NUMEROUS DIETS, THERE ARE MANY FORMS OF fasting, as well. Fasting is usually associated with abstaining from all food and drinks, except for water. But in modern times, intermittent fasting, or IF, has become the dominant fasting practice, since it is easy to do for many people and it provides results that many are looking for. In addition, IF can be implemented into most people's lifestyles and easily become a habit that can improve health and keep weight in check.

However, even IF has various versions that are each effective in their own way. For example, some types of fasting such as 16/8 are more effective at weight loss because they better fit with a person's schedule or comfort level. Other types of IF, such as One Meal a Day, have fans that feel it brings them increased mental clarity and focus. To enjoy the benefits of any healthy dietary change, you have to be able to stick with it and use it as a long-term tool, because health improvements take time.

At the same time, different types of fasting will provide different results. For example, water fasting is often used for medical purposes or to quickly subdue cravings while intermittent fasting seems to be the most beneficial for long-term weight loss. Some types of fasting are done for spiritual or religious purposes, but can serve as a health reset, as well.

No matter what plan you choose, if it is your first time fasting or it has been a while since you have completed a fast, begin with shorter times. This may help to experiment with different fasting windows and to check your energy levels. Then, you can use this information to determine how the fast of your choice will fit in with your commitments and regular schedule.

Intermittent fasts are the safest to perform for beginners while longer fasts may have to be monitored by a health professional that you trust. You can also choose to attend a fasting retreat, which is becoming very popular.

Lastly, if you are on medications, you must check with your prescribing doctor before beginning any fast. The following are descriptions of various types of fasting along with the benefits, drawbacks, and how to do it. This guide can help you decide what kind of fast might be right for you, your schedule, and your goals.

Water Fasting

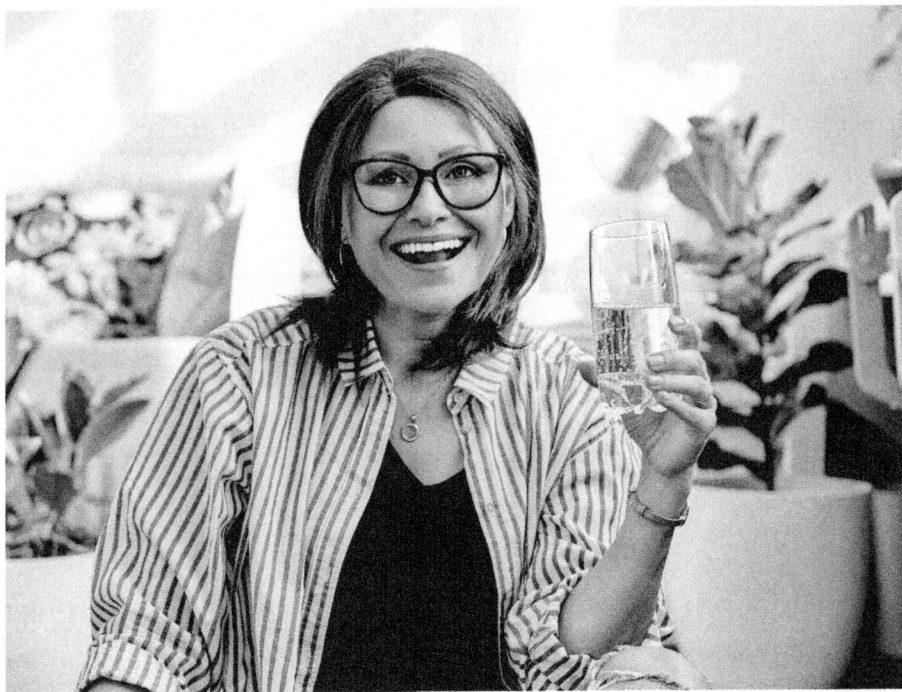

What is it? Water fasting is exactly what it sounds like; you simply abstain from eating and drink water only for a period of time, which can be hours or days. Water fasting is one of the easiest ways to fast and many believe it is the quickest way to achieve results. However, this may be truer for people who have prepared their bodies for a fast (this info will be in a later chapter).

This type of fasting is often performed for religious or spiritual reasons and sometimes for medical reasons, for example in preparation for surgery or medical testing. At the same time, water fasting is one of the quickest ways to induce autophagy and activate the body's self-detoxification processes. This may be why this type of fast has been linked to reducing the risk of diabetes, cancers, and heart disease.

How To: Water fasting seems easy to do at first; simply abstain from food and all beverages except for water. But there are some guidelines to follow to ensure your water fast is performed safely. First and foremost, if you take any medications or are under the care of a doctor, check with that doctor before embarking on any fasting program.

If you begin your fast without preparation, you risk experiencing more side effects, such as headaches and nausea. Therefore, begin your preparation by deciding on which days you will fast. Choose days that will not require a lot of brain power or physical energy, especially if you have never fasted before. Keep track of your diet in the days leading up to the fast and begin implementing certain changes, such as cutting down on grains and sugar for about 4-7 days before you begin your fast. Definitely, cut out junk food for at least a week before you begin, and be sure to drink pure filtered or spring water instead of other beverages.

Since water fasting is more extreme, your body will go into autophagy much quicker than with other types of fasting, especially after the first day. If you have been eating junk food up until your fast, your body will begin to remove that waste first. This means that if you do a 24-hour fast, you may only accomplish detoxing the last few meals. But, if you abstain from junk food and eat healthy, wholesome foods for at least a week before your fast, your body will have a jump start on removing waste and you will have more energy even as cleansing takes place on a deeper level.

Once you begin your fast, abstain from food and drink only fresh, clean water. Drink only 5-10 ounces at a time throughout the day, as needed. Of course, if you are in a very hot and/or humid environment, try to drink more water. Abstain from exercising or exercise at a lowered pace and intensity. If you are very restless, try slow-paced walking, gentle yoga, and gentle stretching. But during a water fast, any intense exercise may burn precious muscle and proteins. Therefore, the best practice is to allow your body to divert the extra energy and resources to detoxification and rebuilding.

After you have completed your first water fast, you will be more prepared to do it again in the future. Water fasting is a practice that many people incorporate for one or two days each week or 3-4 consecutive days each month. The choice is yours and it is perfectly okay to play around with the amount of time you do it. Consistency in this practice is key for best results, while longer fasting times should be supervised by a trusted doctor or health practitioner who can check your vitals and monitor your health.

Breaking a water fast should be done slowly and deliberately. Your digestive processes have not been working for a while and will not just jump back into action. Focus on breaking your fast with plain yogurt, some fruit or a small serving of broth, soup or steamed vegetables. Your first meal can include a small portion of animal protein and vegetables. Be sure to chew the food thoroughly, which sends messages to the rest of your digestive processes to get ready to work. Pay attention and stop eating when you are full or satiated.

What are the Benefits: There are numerous benefits to water fasting, especially if you have properly prepared yourself. In the medical world, water fasting is often recommended to patients before chemotherapy treatment as a way to lessen uncomfortable side effects. But not only that, it turns out that fasting for 48 hours slowed the growth and spread of certain cancers.[10] Most people reading this will not have tumors or cancer, however, any of our cells have the ability to become cancerous. Since it is unlikely that we will be tested for cancer on a regular basis, taking precautions to prevent future diseases cannot hurt.

Weight loss is another benefit touted with water fasting. The key is to first prepare your body for fasting, then have a set meal plan for after the fast. Having a healthy plan surrounding your water fast and sticking to it will lead to long-term weight loss, and can help change your eating habits, making it easier to keep the weight off. You will find that you'll naturally crave healthier foods after a fast.

Moreover, fasting for 24 hours enhances human growth hormone (HGH) secretion. In fact, one study at the Intermountain Medical Center (Horne, Anderson 2011) found that HGH production increased about 1300% on average for women and almost 2,000% for men! This is important since HGH supports brain health, tissue repair (like muscle building after a workout), and thermogenesis (fat burning), and helps boost metabolism.

Water fasting is very beneficial to help bring your appetite under control. Many people feel that going on a water fast for 1-3 days helps get them back on track with a diet, overcome plateaus, and

---

10   Lee C, Raffaghello L, Brandhorst S, et al. Fasting cycles retard growth of tumors and sensitize a range of cancer cell types to chemotherapy. Science translational medicine 2012;4:124ra27.

greatly reduce cravings that may begin to creep in. The following are more benefits found with water fasting:

- HGH production
- Improvement of liver function to help burn stored fat and fatty buildup
- Hunger regulation and reduction of cravings
- Improvement of cardiovascular health when used regularly
- Preservation of memory and improvement of cognitive function
- Lower blood pressure
- Stabilization of blood sugar

Of course, each of the above benefits depends upon how you use water fasting, for example, how many days you fast. Other factors that will determine your benefits include your level of health at the beginning of the fast and if you are on any medications. Moreover, you will be able to see how well and how long you prepared for your fast, and what you should do afterward.

If you have never done a water fast in the past, I feel the best approach for most is to incorporate short fasts of 12 to 18 hours and if you do well, go for 24 hours. As your health improves, then try for longer water fasts, but with longer preparation so you get the most benefits for your hard work.

What are the drawbacks? As with any dietary practice, there may be drawbacks to water fasting. These include excessive weight loss for those who embark on an extended fast, orthostatic hypotension, which is a sudden drop of blood pressure when you stand up too quickly, and increased amounts of uric acid in your blood (due to your body detoxing), which can lead to gout flare-ups.

Water fasts are difficult for those who have never fasted and might trigger extreme hunger, headaches, and nausea. If you do not drink enough water, you risk dehydration, which happens to some people who are not accustomed to drinking water throughout the day. And of course, it is not good for those with certain medical conditions or medications.

Who should not do it:

- People who take medications should always work with their doctor before any diet changes, especially fasting. Water fasting may be dangerous for people on blood pressure medications.
- People with an eating disorder, as it could trigger more issues.
- People with diabetes should talk to their doctors first and have medical supervision during a water fast (if the doctor approves that fasting is okay). They can also choose to work with Dr. Fung in Canada who specializes in water fasting programs for diabetics.
- Women who are pregnant or breastfeeding should not do a water fast. They need extra nutrition for this time to support all of their bodily changes as it gets ready for the baby, and of course, the baby needs nutrition. This is also not the time for detoxing.
- People with eating disorders should not try water fasting.

Intermittent Fasting or IF

What is it? Intermittent fasting (IF) is an easy and effective way to fast for many people. It is based on fasting "intermittently," or at intervals. The fasting interval may be an entire 24-hour period once or more each week, or maybe 12 hours or more each day. The time that you are not fasting is often referred to as the "feeding window" and it is usually set with some regularity, making it easier to follow.

Some experts believe that IF is natural because our ancestors survived on hunting, which often resulted in feasts or famine. Some also believe that to stop eating at dark is natural, since our ancestors did not have electricity, so chances are they slept during darkness. Moreover, they survived during these long bouts of not eating while having to continuously hunt, create shelter, forage, and take care of their families.

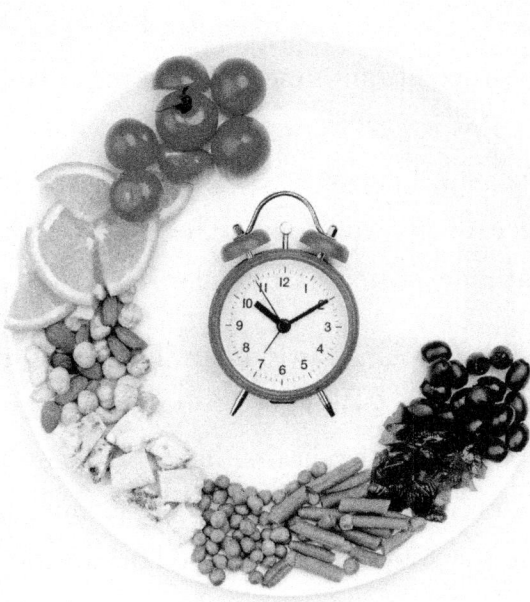

In today's culture, it is common to consume too many calories while partaking in less activity thanks to television, the internet, and other forms of entertainment that breed inactivity. However, IF has proven to provide numerous, seemingly natural health benefits such as improved blood pressure and heart rate. It seems to trigger a metabolic switch that puts our entire body into a healthier, more protective mode.

Intermittent fasting focuses more on when to eat as opposed to the actual food or diet. Some advocates claim that you can eat anything you want, but logic should dictate that when restricting your food choices in any way, healthy food should make up most of your meals. Following a Mediterranean diet, Keto diet, or other healthy options will provide the best results.

How to: There are a few different ways to incorporate IF into your lifestyle. Each program provides benefits of weight loss, improved heart health, improved brain function, and improved blood sugar levels. However, this is also dependent upon what you eat during your feeding window, how well you stick with the program, and your level of health when you begin. The following are the various ways to follow an intermittent fasting plan.

12/12 and 16/8 fasting plans are similar. The first number is how many hours to fast in a 24-hour period and the second number is the number of consecutive hours that food is consumed during the same 24 hours; some refer to this as the feeding window. Most people begin the fast sometime before bed or around dark, so they sleep through most of the fasting period. This makes the plan easier to follow with less temptation.

For example, if you follow the 12/12 fasting plan, you will fast for 12 hours and eat any meals and snacks during the other 12 hours. Your day might look like this:

- Begin your fast at 7 pm and do not eat or drink anything other than water or tea again until after 7 am, at which time you may have a cup of coffee or tea with milk or a smoothie.
- Consume healthy meals and beverages until 7 pm and then fast again. During your fasting time, only drink water, black coffee, or herbal tea with no sweeteners, cream, milk, or other additives.
- Of course, you can fast from 7 pm to 7 am, 8 pm to 8 am, or even 4 pm to 4 am, if that fits your schedule.
- 16/8 is the most popular fasting time for weight loss, and many experts advise that for best weight loss results, one should stop eating at 2 pm. Your day would look like this:
- Begin your fast at 2 pm and drink only water or herbal tea until 6 am the next day, at which time you can have a beverage with added milk or coconut oil and breakfast.
- Consume only healthy meals, snacks, and beverages until 2 pm, and then abstain from food (fast) again until the next morning at 6 am.

As above, your feeding window and fasting time should accommodate your schedule, so if it is easier for you to eat from 9 am to 5 pm and then fast from 5 pm until 11 am the next day, then go for it. You will still reap the benefits.

24-hour fasting is another popular way to do IF, which is common among many religious sects. It requires one 24-hour period of fasting in which only water is consumed, once per week. Most people do not follow a strict 24 hours, but instead, simply wake up, live their day without eating, go to bed and then resume eating when they awake the next day. This type of fasting has shown incredible long-term benefits like improved brain health and cardiovascular health, but of course, this is dependent upon what you do the other six days of the week.

What are the Benefits? The main benefit of IF is how easy it can be. Some people who need to build discipline may begin a schedule of IF and start by not being overly strict with their food choices. As time goes on and results are seen, such as fewer cravings and a more controlled appetite, it may become easier to make healthier food choices while giving up sweets or junk food altogether.

Evidentially, IF seems to be the most studied type of fasting, therefore has more research backing it than other forms of fasting. Note that this does not make other types of fasting less beneficial, just based more on historical as well as anecdotal evidence. The research backing up IF shows that IF is beneficial for fat loss, blood sugar levels, improved heart health, and even improved brain health. Check out the following.

- **Fast Loss:** Overwhelming evidence, both scientific and anecdotal, show that nearly all forms of IF result in weight loss. But what about actual fat loss? Apparently so. In one study published in the Journal of Translational Medicine, it was found that eight weeks of following the 16/8 IF plan resulted in decreased fat mass and improved health biomarkers when done with resistance training.[11] While this is only one study (there are more) IF also seems to improve the output of human growth hormone, which helps regulate adipose tissue (fat).

- **Lower Blood Pressure:** Quite often, when the diet is improved, overall health improves. But IF may be one of the easiest ways to help take control of your blood pressure. A 2018 study published in the Journal of Nutrition and Healthy Aging reported that 16/8 fasting lowered blood pressure in obese patients.[12] While these were only short-term results, one can probably experience long-term ones if very healthy foods were consumed during the feeding window, along with other lifestyle changes, such as stopping smoking or reduced alcohol consumption.

- **Stem Cell Regeneration:** Following IF plans, which limit the feeding window to 8 hours or less for at least 21 days, results in not only weight loss, but also in the enhancement of stem cell regeneration. Besides, it can result in long-lasting improved metabolic effects.[13] Stem cells serve as part of our bodies' repair system and may develop into a number of different cells throughout the body, including cells in the muscle and brain tissue.

- **Autophagy:** Intermittent fasting provides a window of opportunity for your body to activate its internal detoxification system known as autophagy. This is when your body regenerates or elim-

11 Moro T, Tinsley G, Bianco A, et al. Effects of eight weeks of time-restricted feeding (16/8) on basal metabolism, maximal strength, body composition, inflammation, and cardiovascular risk factors in resistance-trained males. J Transl Med. 2016;14(1):290. Published 2016 Oct 13. doi:10.1186/s12967-016-1044-0

12 Gabel, Kelsey et al. 'Effects of 8-hour Time Restricted Feeding on Body Weight and Metabolic Disease Risk Factors in Obese Adults: A Pilot Study'. 1 Jan. 2018 : 345 – 353.

13 Mattson MP, Longo VD, Harvie M. Impact of intermittent fasting on health and disease processes. Ageing Res Rev. 2017 Oct;39:46-58. doi: 10.1016/j.arr.2016.10.005. Epub 2016 Oct 31. PMID: 2/810402; PMCID: PMC5411330.

inates damaged cells and begins anywhere from 6-12 hours after fasting begins.

What are the drawbacks? The major drawback of IF is similar to dieting, but to a lesser extreme. While 95% of diets fail, meaning the dieter either quits or gains the weight back, it seems that a research study published in the Journal of the American Medical Association (JAMA) Internal medicine to study the effects of restricted calories led to a 38% dropout rate for those using IF. This suggests that fasting may be a pitfall for some, however, 38% is still much better than 95%! If you tried IF and had any success, there is no reason to not try it again; you may get it right with practice.

Another drawback of IF is the encouragement of some experts who claim you can eat anything you want. This leads some people to believe they can eat more calories during the feeding window and still see results. Unfortunately, at least one recent study showed that simply using IF by cramming an unhealthy diet into the feeding window with no change in calories resulted in very few changes in health or weight.[14]

Who should not do it: While the benefits are numerous and implementing it is fairly easy, IF is not for everyone.

• Women who are pregnant or breastfeeding should not fast because during this time your body needs around-the-clock nutrition to feed the baby (both while pregnant and nursing).

---

14   Lowe DA, Wu N, Rohdin-Bibby L, et al. Effects of Time-Restricted Eating on Weight Loss and Other Metabolic Parameters in Women and Men With Overweight and Obesity: The TREAT Randomized Clinical Trial. JAMA Intern Med. 2020;180(11):1491–1499. doi:10.1001/jamainternmed.2020.4153

- People who are underweight or struggle to gain weight should try other dietary health methods, as fasting can lead to more weight loss.
- Most people under 18 can often use other options to regain health, since the body is still developing, therefore needs nutrition to continue a healthy development. With that being said, if someone under 18 truly needs to lose weight, check with your doctor before embarking on any type of diet, especially fasting.

Protein Sparing Modified Fast (PSMF)

What is it? The Protein Sparing Modified Fast was made popular by my friend, Maria Emmerich, the Queen of the Keto Diet. PSMF is a tool designed to kick-start rapid weight loss by minimizing carbs and fat while supplying the body with adequate protein. This approach mimics the rapid weight loss benefits of fasting while preventing the loss of lean mass.

The PSMF was first introduced in the 1970s to help people with obesity lose weight under the guidance of a physician. It is a very low-calorie diet designed to aid weight loss and preserve muscle mass. Originally, it was performed for 4-6 months in a clinical setting. Today, we have a modified version of this fast that should be used occasionally when an additional boost to one's weight loss efforts is needed.

How to: The PSMF consists of fewer than 800 calories per day. These calories come from lean proteins, such as fish, chicken, pork, or egg whites. You can also add some non-starchy vegetables like broccoli, leafy greens, cabbage, cauliflower, mushrooms, Brussels sprouts, celery, tomatoes, and onions.

It is recommended that you consume 1.2-1.5 grams of protein per kilogram of your goal body weight per day. For example, a person whose goal weight is 150 lbs (68 kgs) would eat 81-102 grams of protein per day.

Carbohydrates should be kept to a minimum and only consume very low-carb veggies like mentioned above.

Fat is limited to whatever is found naturally in the lean protein. Added fats of any kind – oils, dressings, spreads, etc., – are not permitted.

PSMF is used for 2-3 days to help overcome weight loss plateaus or to quickly get into ketosis. Some people do 2-3 days every week in order to lose weight more quickly. It is not advisable to follow the PSMF 7 days a week. Three days a week is safe to do, the other 4 days will act like a refeeding phase to keep you not only satiated but nourished. While there are no essential carbohydrates, fat is crucial for all bodily functions so it's not advisable to eliminate them from our diet in the long term. Make sure that you are eating plenty of healthy fats on your refeeding days.

What are the Benefits? This fast is called "protein sparing" because it is designed to preserve your muscle. Some believe that longer water fasts can lead to some muscle loss so PSMF can help avoid this issue while still providing most of the benefits of fasting. For this reason, this type of fasting is very popular with bodybuilders as well.

In addition to weight loss, PSMF also helps lower inflammation and bloating. You will likely notice that you're urinating a lot more frequently on your fasting days.

What are the drawbacks? Because you are eating zero fat and carbs, PSMF can leave you feeling hungry and low on energy. If you're not starting the diet already in ketosis, it can be a bit challenging as your body adjusts. You may experience headaches, nausea, and lightheadedness. Make sure to add a little pinch of pink Himalayan salt to your water to help with these issues.

Eating only protein can be a bit boring, especially when you're used to eating a wide variety of foods. Maria Emmerich offers some great PSMF recipes on her website and I highly recommend her cookbooks as well.

Who should not do it: PSMF is not suitable for anyone already at a healthy weight. Those with eating disorders and pregnant or nursing women should also avoid PSMF. If you have a serious health condition, please check with your medical provider first.

> **FAST FACT**
>
> Studies on rats and a small group of people in a clinical trial show that fasting while on chemotherapy helps to protect white blood cells and also grow new ones.

Juice Fasting

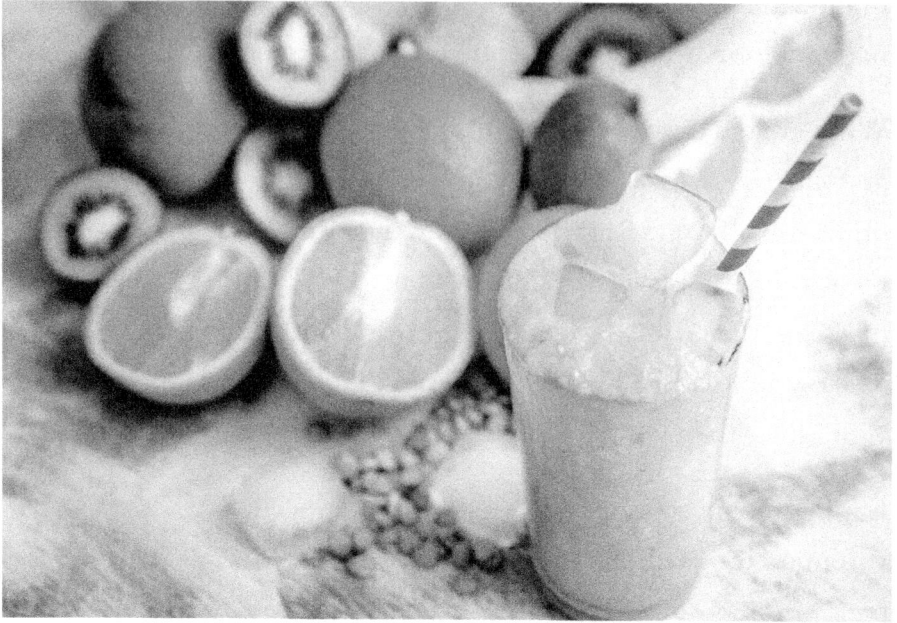

Juice fasting is similar to water fasting, but with a daily intake of fresh-made vegetable or vegetable and fruit juice mixtures as sustenance. Making fresh juice as part of a health plan is often used today for healing, and it became popular with Norman Walker, a health advocate and pioneer in vegetable juice for healing and health. In fact, his book, *Fresh Vegetable and Fruit Juices* published in 1936 lists a number of ailments, what type of juice would promote healing, and then the nutritional information of why.

Since then, juicing has become popular among many health advocates. Stores sell bottled vegetable juice and even mainstream food corporations may add some type of vegetable to their once 100% fruit juice, while fresh-made vegetable juice can be purchased at many health food stores and restaurants.

What is it? Juice fasting is the act of abstaining from solid foods and replacing meals with fresh juice, instead. The type of juice used depends on the person and how often one drinks depends on one's health goals and level of health. Mainly, juice fasting is used to cleanse and detoxify the body, lose weight, or both.

Juice fasting is different than simply replacing food with blended fruits and vegetables or smoothies. Juicing removes the pulp of the foods so all that is left is what some refer to as the "mineral water" of the produce. It can be high in calories and sugar, and with no fiber or pulp to slow the absorption, a juice program should be planned ahead of time so you can evaluate how much sugar is consumed.

Drinking vegetable juice provides your body with more nutrients and enzymes than water fasting or eating the same foods, as nutrients can be left in the fiber instead of absorbed. At the same time, most people cannot digest as many vegetables as they can drink. When you drink vegetables and fruits without the fiber, nutrients are absorbed instead of digested, so you get full advantage of their properties. But juicing can stimulate your body to detoxify quicker, which can lead to detox side effects like nausea or headache. If mild, these will often pass on their own and possibly quicker by drinking pure water.

How to: To do a juice fast, first plan out in advance which days you will do your fast. The most common lengths of time are 1 – 3 days while some people may go as long as 30 days (but not normally recommended without supervision).

Planning should also include how many calories you want to consume, and which juices you drink. For a well-rounded blend of nutrients, use a mixture of leafy greens, a small amount of root vegetables such as beetroot, some herbs like ginger root, garlic, turmeric root, or even cayenne, and small amounts of fruit. If you are unsure of which ones to use, some popular combinations include:

- ½ apple, kale, 3 carrots, 5 celery stalks, ¼ inch of turmeric root
- 4 carrots, ¼ inch of ginger root, juice of ½ lemon and ¼ beetroot
- A handful of greens of choice, peach slices, mint leaves, 4-5 celery stalks

Some common vegetables and their uses include:

- Beetroots for liver support
- Carrots for skin and eyes
- Celery for a healthy heart

When planning your juice, keep in mind that more is not always better. As you see above, one of the recipes calls for only ¼ beetroot. This is because as beneficial as this veggie can be for your liver, it contains oxalic acid, which can be detrimental to the kidneys and joints when consumed in high amounts. This is yet another reason to plan your juices for each day.

It is best to use organic produce as fresh as possible whenever possible It is also helpful to plan out your day according to which juice you will have and at what time. This will help you stay on track and take the guesswork out of what to drink next. You can also use your plan to help you shop. It is easiest to stick with the same juice each day, but not necessary.

Be sure to drink water throughout the day, and it is okay to have herbal tea. Some people prefer to consume bone broth each day, especially for fasts lasting longer than one day, to ensure adequate protein and nutrient intake.

If you do not have a juicer of your own, find a local store to buy fresh juice from. Fresh juice is best when consumed within 30 minutes of being made to take advantage of the live enzymes. Bottled vegetable juice does not offer much in the way of nutrition and is devoid of enzymes, so best avoided. Adding a green superfood powder, such as barley grass or spirulina, is beneficial for some.

Before you begin, prepare your body by eating lighter and consuming only healthy foods for at least four days before your fast. When you begin, drink water and at least 3-6 glasses of vegetable juice per day and whatever you need to fulfill your caloric requirements. If you don't count calories, at least drink four, 10-ounce glasses of juice for the nutrients. If you have to drink it in 3 due to time constraints, that's okay. Some people prefer to make their juice for the entire day all at once, then divide it out throughout the day. While you will still benefit from your fast, you may get more benefits from fresh juice since the enzymes are available only for the first 30 minutes or so.

What are the Benefits? The benefits of drinking vegetable juice will vary greatly, depending on if you drink fresh or bottled juice, how much you drink, how long you fast, and how well you prepared for the fast. Most people enjoy weight loss (mainly temporary if not followed through with a healthy diet), more energy, improved digestion, and improved skin tone.

One study set out to prove that a three-day vegetable and fruit juice fast improved the gut microbiome, which is linked to digestion, metabolism, and overall health. During this study, of 20 healthy adults, healthy bacteria in the gut microbiome increased and thus altered the microbiota to be favorable to weight loss. Each participant consumed six, 16-ounce bottles of juice with greens, beetroot, citrus, cayenne, and vanilla almond. Each showed a significant decrease in weight and body mass index.[15] This is exciting, considering fresh juice with live enzymes should show even greater improvements in health.

Along with weight loss and digestive benefits, a juice fast can boost blood nutrient levels such as vitamin C, beta carotene, and folate. In addition, the body can stock up on the many micronutrients that are part of any vegetable and fruit's nutrient package, which are often not part of vitamin and/or mineral supplements.

Since juice improves digestion, a juice cleanse can help your body cleanse and detoxify. Since energy will not be needed for digestion, your body can use the energy for detoxification processes like autophagy. And the effects may be amplified since you are consuming even more nutrients and enzymes.

Anecdotal evidence includes benefits such as healthier-looking skin with more glow, improved energy, improved hair texture, and even stronger eyesight. Juice fasting for short periods of time can improve health, but for most people, do not work out long term.

What are the drawbacks? One drawback of juice fasting is the extra-strong detoxing process. Sometimes the body is not ready to simply give up eating and focus all its energies on healing and de-

---

15   Henning SM, Yang J, Shao P, et al. Health benefit of vegetable/fruit juice-based diet: Role of microbiome. Sci Rep. 2017;7(1):2167. Published 2017 May 19. doi:10.1038/s41598-017-02200-6

toxification. This can take a toll on the body with some unexpected consequences such as blood sugar dips and spikes from fasting and then excessive sugar consumption if too many beetroots or carrots are consumed.

Having to make or obtain fresh-made juice each day can be time-consuming, or expensive if you purchase juice already made. Restrictions such as these eventually become obstacles for many, which means a greater chance of not following through.

Then there's the issue of oxalates. Oxalates are substances that bind to calcium and are also known as nephrotoxins, or substances that are toxic to the kidneys. Unfortunately, some healthy foods that are often used in juicing contain oxalates, and drinking their juice can lead to oxalate overload. When this happens, you may notice aching in your neck or areas that are prone to arthritis or may feel pain in the kidneys. Problems take place when juice fasting is done for long periods of time, or when too much juice with vegetables containing oxalates is consumed. Some of these foods include:

• Spinach
• Swiss chard
• Rhubarb
• Okra
• Leeks
• Beets

Because of the above issues with calories, sugar, and oxalates, juice fasting is best done only short-term. The difficulty of keeping track of your intake, nutrient intake, and the process of making or obtaining the juice can become difficult for most schedules. Therefore, if you do a juice fast, proceed with caution and remember it is a temporary health boost that should be followed by a long-term health plan.

Who should not do it:

- Because of the above-explained risks, those with arthritis or any arthritic conditions should avoid juice fasting and find an alternative, such as intermittent fasting with perhaps a few glasses of vegetable juice each week if tolerated
- Diabetics should avoid juice fasts due to sugar spikes. If you really want to try one, or drink fresh vegetable and/or fruit juices, always check with your doctor, first.
- Those with kidney disease or any kidney problems should avoid juice fasting.
- As always, pregnant or nursing women should not juice fast.

Master Cleanse

The Master Cleanse is sometimes referred to as the lemonade cleanse, the lemonade diet or the lemonade fast. Created in 1941 by Stanley Burroughs, this fast has very specific protocols and recipes that are to be used to help the body cleanse and detoxify.

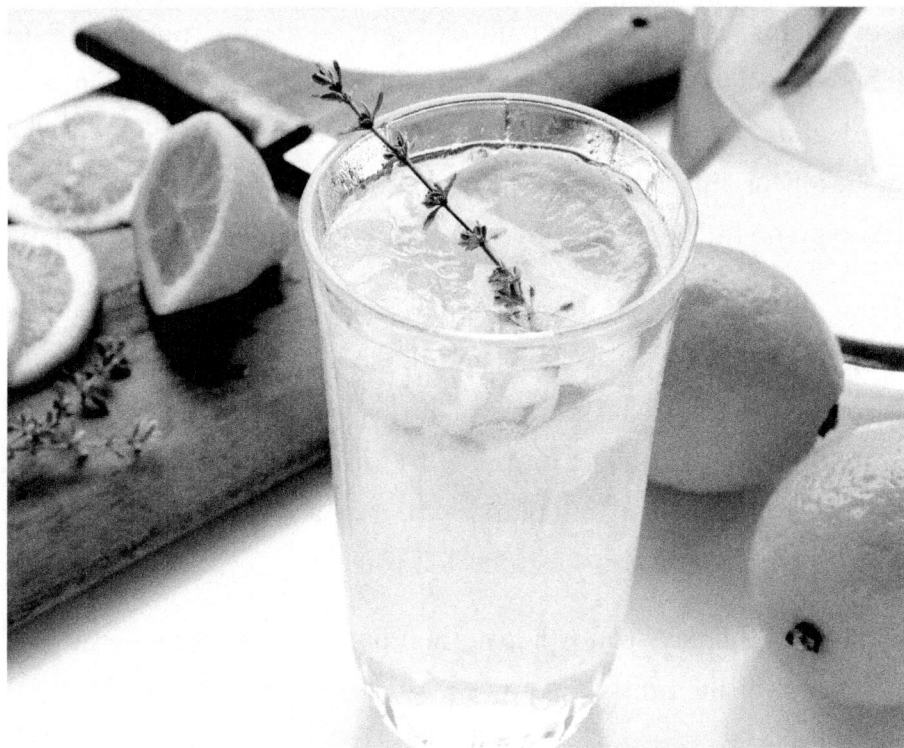

This fasting cleanse had a resurgence thanks to celebrities like Beyonce who claim it helped them shed weight and feel better. At the same time, there is much criticism for being overly restrictive and can even cause the purging of essential nutrients along with toxins.

What is it? The Master Cleanse is a 10-day fast in which you abstain from all food and drinks except water, the specialized "lemonade" drink, and saltwater or a laxative. There is a leading-in period (what I refer to as preparing your body) and a post-period where you gradually reintroduce food. In the book, The Master Cleanser, Mr. Burroughs recommends going back to a plant-based diet with very little dairy products or meat.

This cleanse is not for the faint of heart, as the instructions are to follow the cleanse precisely or you will have complications including feeling sick, fatigued, and achy with cravings. Because of the inclusion of salt water or a laxative, many advocates who do this fast plan on little activity and may even take off work for a few days.

How to: Some preparation is required for this fast, and should be adhered to for the best results and the least side effects. The fast is meant to last for 10 days, however, if this is your first time, it may be a good idea to shorten it to three or four days to "test the waters." At the same time, you can plan for 10 days and know that it is okay to stop at any time your instincts tell you.

First, plan the days you will fast, then purchase the ingredients you will need for the prep days and the drink, which include:

- Fresh lemons for freshly squeezed lemon juice
- Organic grade B maple syrup (no imitations or cheap syrups, as this syrup provides nutrients)
- Ground cayenne pepper
- Filtered water
- Epsom salt or an over-the-counter herbal laxative

Prepare your body by doing the following:

- **Day 1:** consume only living, raw foods like vegetables, fruits, and sprouts
- **Day 2:** Drink only soup broths and vegetable juice
- **Day 3:** Drink only orange juice, freshly squeezed, organic juice is best

On day four you will begin the Master Cleanse fasting phase, in which you will consume the specialized "lemonade" drinks from 6 – 12 times each day, or when you feel hungry. The recipe is as follows:

- 2 Tbsp freshly squeezed, organic lemon juice
- 2 Tbsp of organic, grade B maple syrup
- 1/10 tsp ground cayenne pepper
- 10 ounces of filtered water

If you choose to take a laxative, take it in the evening. If you choose the saltwater flush, drink it first thing in the morning. The saltwater flush is made by dissolving 2 teaspoons of pink Himalayan salt (or another non-iodized sea salt) into four cups of warm water. Lemon juice can be added for flavor if needed. The entire mixture must be drunk on an empty stomach, first thing in the morning, as quickly as possible (without harming yourself, of course).

Follow this protocol for 10 days (or for as long as you choose to) and then do the following to ease out of the fast:

- **Day 1:** Drink only freshly squeezed, organic orange juice throughout the day
- **Day 2:** Consume only soup broths and vegetable juice in small amounts, throughout the day
- **Day 3:** Consume only living foods spread out into small meals or snacks
- Day 4 and after, slowly reintroduce healthy foods in small meals until you are eating regular meals. Focus on whole, healthy foods with plenty of protein to help feed your muscles and rebuild any lost tissue.

What are the Benefits? The most reported benefit of this cleanse is weight loss. Keep in mind it will be temporary as most weight will come back when you begin eating since it was mainly water weight (fluids) loss. However, phasing back into a healthy lifestyle with a healthy diet will help you to continue to lose weight in the long term.

Improved digestion is reported by many fans of the Master Cleanse. This may be due to a combination of things such as abstaining from food, which allows digestive enzymes to rest and reset, and removing toxins that can throw off the balance of the gut microbiome.

While the fast can be draining for some, those who are experienced with it feel they have more energy at certain times throughout the cleanse, but mainly feel renewed afterward. Clearing waste and toxins from the body can definitely have this effect, as the body clears waste from the brain area, as well. But again, this feeling will last only as long as you continue to eat healthily.

Some of the ingredients of the Master Cleanse are very beneficial and have positive health implications. Vitamin C from lemon juice is a powerful antioxidant that can improve skin tone and even promote thermogenesis, or a rise in metabolic heat, which improves the body's ability to burn fat. Organic maple syrup has a lower GI score than other sugars and is used to help with blood sugar issues during the fast. (Whether this works or not is individual and if you take medications for blood pressure, only do this with your doctor's permission to stay safe.) But maple syrup also contains powerful nutrients that can help lower inflammation, improve skin, and provide important minerals like potassium, zinc, magnesium, and calcium.

What are the drawbacks? Drawbacks of this fast include the typical side effects that accompany most fasting and detoxification programs. However, they may feel more intensified because of the drink and laxative/salt water flush. These symptoms include headaches, fatigue, nausea, dizziness, bad breath, cramping, and dehydration if you are not consuming enough water.

Some health experts believe following a protocol of fasting and purging may encourage eating disorders for some people. Also, because of the laxative or purging effect, this cleanse may cause an electrolyte imbalance, which can cause dizziness and even fainting.

Who should not do it: There are certain groups of people who should avoid this cleanse, such as:

- Those with diabetes or other blood sugar issues should discuss any diet changes, especially fasting, with their doctor.
- People with cancer, anemia, and other serious medical issues should talk with their doctor or skip this cleanse altogether.
- Those who are underweight should not embark on this cleanse.
- People with or who are prone to eating disorders should avoid this cleanse.
- Pregnant or nursing mothers.

Fat Fast

Fat and fast are not terms that are normally used together, and in the case of a fat fast, things get even stranger. Fat fasting is a technique used by many people to lose fat, and while it sounds counterintuitive, it actually works. But this technique or fast is only ef-

FAST FACT

In animals, studies show fasting protects the brain from damage after a stroke and speeds recovery.

fective when used for 2 − 5 days and any longer than this will cause muscle loss and other issues that will sabotage weight loss.

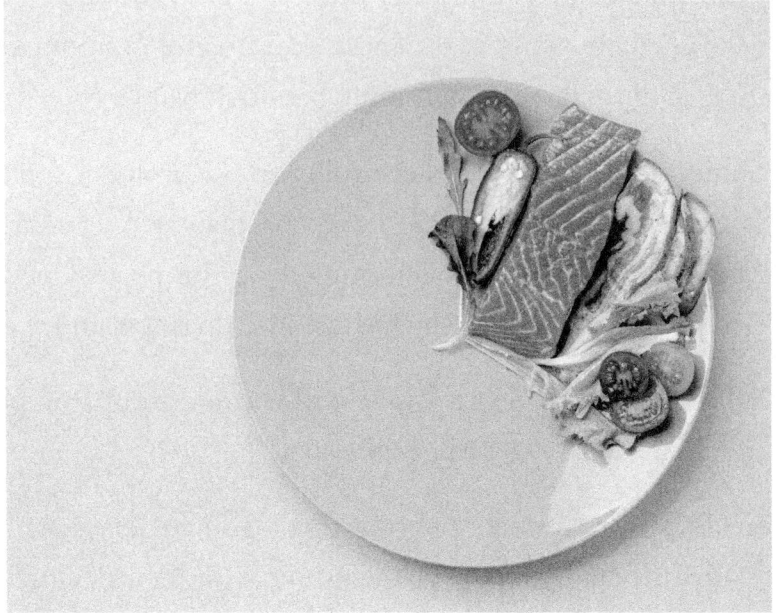

This fast is intended to help people lose weight by stimulating ketosis, or the process of burning fat for fuel. But it is used in very specific situations such as for people who are on a diet plateau of two weeks or longer and for those who need to stimulate ketosis quickly. It is not to be used long-term or consistently.

During a fat fast, very few calories from carbohydrates and proteins are consumed, with the bulk of calories coming from fat. This forces the body into a state called lipolysis, in which it burns fat stores for fuel. During lipolysis, fats are converted to triglycerides, into glycerol, and then fatty acids which the liver then uses to create ketones which are used as fuel. This is called ketosis.

The process of lipolysis will not take place when we eat foods that are converted into glucose, which is normally the body's main source of energy. But excluding carbs and proteins from your diet leaves very little else for the body to burn as fuel so fat becomes the main source of energy and the goal of low-carb and keto diets.

What is it? Fat fasting is not true fasting, as the goal is to consume between 1,000 and 1,200 calories per day, with 80%–90% of those calories being from fat. The meals are broken down into small portions to include 4 – 5 meals a day, making it easier for the liver to do its job. As mentioned, the fat fast is done for 2 – 5 days, with the average being 3 days, since it is very restrictive.

The goal of a fat fast is not weight loss over the fasting days, but to stimulate ketosis for long-term weight loss. You may lose up to 8 pounds in three days, but at least half will be regained as you start eating again. If you choose to do this fast, look for lasting results and use this only periodically to help stimulate ketosis when you hit a plateau. Some people use this technique after a cheat day or after a vacation to get them back on track.

How to: Doing a fat fast is relatively simple to follow, but you do need some recipes on hand to help you stay on track and control your caloric intake as well as macronutrient balance. Determine your desired daily caloric intake and divide that up into 4-5 "meals," but keep in mind the meals may not be a true meal, but instead a beverage with coconut butter or heavy cream as the source of calories.

For people who need to eat 4-5 times a day, then fat bomb recipes will help you create a menu.

The following are each considered a meal during a fat fast, and 4-5 of these would normally be consumed in the course of a day. Of course, you would have to adjust the amounts, so you meet your personal caloric requirements.

- Coffee with ¼ cup of heavy cream or 1 Tbsp of coconut oil
- 3 slices of bacon
- ½ avocado topped with 1 tsp olive oil, salt & pepper
- 1 ounce Macadamia nuts
- 2 ounces of cream cheese with 1 celery stalk
- Small beef burger on 1 small piece of butter lettuce with 1 tsp mustard or mayo
- 1 cup of chicken broth with 2 Tbsp of heavy cream
- 3 slices of bacon with 2 egg yolks cooked in the bacon grease
- 2 servings of sugar-free Jello with ¼ cup of whipped cream
- 4 ounces of sliced mushrooms sauteed in 1 Tbsp of butter and topped with 1 Tbsp cream cheese
- Salad with 100g tomatoes, 80g feta cheese, 80 grams green olives, 1 Tbsp olive oil and herbs such as basil

Fat bombs are mini meals that are often made in batches and stored for meals. Creating a few batches of fat bombs can result in easy grab-and-go meals during your fat fast. Recipes include mini portions of mixtures like salmon and cream cheese balls, sausage, egg and cheese "muffins," and pizza bombs with mozzarella cheese, bacon, and tomato bits. There are numerous recipes online and making a few ahead of your fast can help you get through it much easier.

Be sure to drink water throughout the day to help you avoid dehydration and help you feel full. You can also drink herbal teas, as long as you do not add sweeteners, sugar, or other additives unless it is part of a meal.

What are the Benefits? The benefits of fat fasting are first and foremost the stimulation of lipolysis and ketosis. It is a quick way to help anyone get their diet back on track and get the body into high fat-burning mode. And while it's not normally used as a way to lose weight, if you do need to lose a few pounds for an upcoming event, you can use a fat fast to help while moving your body into ketosis at the same time.

Breaking through weight loss plateaus is what the fat fast was initially created for by Dr. Robert Atkins. It can be frustrating for anyone who works hard to stick with a diet plan only to stop losing weight a couple of months into it. But the fat fast is a strategy that can be used to move your body back into ketosis or to take your body into a deeper level of ketosis so you can get back to reaching your goals.

Ketosis is the goal and best benefit of doing a fat fast. Burning fat is healthy for your body and your brain, and one major ketone called BHB may be a more efficient brain fuel that stimulates increased cerebral blood flow. This can help protect your brain from certain neurological diseases as you continue to lose weight. So, it seems helping your body go into a state of ketosis can result in a thinner and smarter you!

What are the drawbacks? The fat fast is to help you get into ketosis quickly, so may have the same symptoms of what some call the keto flu. The symptoms range from headaches to chills and mild nausea, but can sometimes be remedied by taking MCT oil, increasing electrolytes, and maintaining hydration.

Because of the quick transition into ketosis, some people may feel fatigued during their fast. The best solution is to relax as often as you can and allow your body to detox and transition. Drink plenty of water, and add a little fresh lemon juice for a pick-me-up and electrolytes. Avoid exercise during the fast, and for those who feel they must exercise, do mild exercise like walking or stretching.

Some experts believe that fat fasting may lead to spikes or unhealthy fluctuations in blood sugar levels or may interfere with hormone levels. However, for the average healthy person, this is often not an issue due to the short amount of time. If you have any concerns or health issues, talk to your doctor before trying a fat fast.

Who should not do it: Simply put, this fast should not be done by people with diabetes or heart disease, pregnant or nursing mothers. If you are on any medications, talk to your doctor before any diet changes or fasting.

Fasting Mimicking Diet

Some people cannot or prefer to not fast. Sometimes health reasons might interfere while others may feel they won't have the energy for their daily commitments. Whatever the reason may be, the fasting mimicking diet (FMD) is a strategy used to "trick" the body into fasting mode.

Developed by Dr. Valter Longo, Ph.D. and director of the Longevity Institute at the University of Southern California, FMD is a low-calorie diet plan that some label as a form of intermittent fasting. The diet is intended to slow the aging process while promoting cell regeneration, which supports tissue repair necessary for healing and longevity. While it is not true fasting, the effects on the body's response are similar to the effects of fasting.

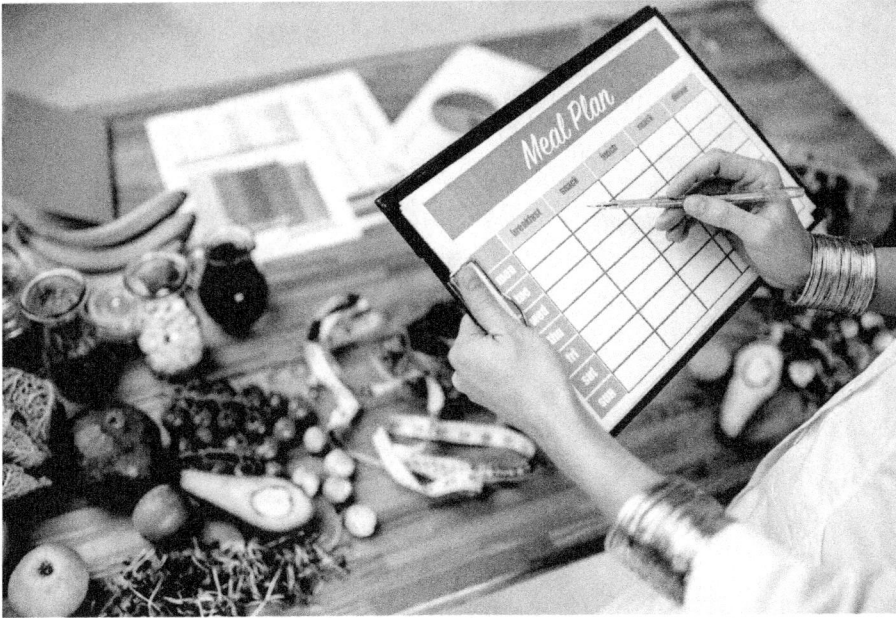

What is it? The fast-mimicking diet is a 5-day, plant-based plan that nutritionally supports the body while providing the same health benefits as fasting. During the program, calories are reduced to about 40% of what an average person would normally consume while proteins come from foods like tempeh, pulses, and tofu. The diet is designed to reduce the risks of fasting such as fatigue, low blood sugar, and low blood pressure.

The program is patented with a specific combination of healthy fats, plant proteins, and low GI carbs and is said to regulate nutrient pathways to cause the cells to act as they would in fasting mode.

A clinical trial led by Dr. Longo showed that participants who followed his FMD lost an average of six pounds, mainly as a reduction of body fat.

There are now keto and low-carb versions of the FMD so you can also modify this fast to fit your dietary needs. For the moment, however, we are focusing on the original version by Dr. Longo.

How to: The studies showing the efficacy of the FMD used the specific food plans created by Dr. Longo. These are sold on his website, ProLon Fast, at a cost of about US $250 for a five-day plan. Included in the daily plan are soup packets, snacks like olives and kale crackers, a nutrition bar, and a specialized glycerol energy drink also intended to preserve muscle mass.

To do the fasting mimicking diet, first purchase the kit from the ProLon website. Next, prepare your body as you would for other fasts, by eating only healthy, clean foods and drinking plenty of water for at least four days. Begin your fast by following the instructions supplied with the meal kits, which is basically to consume the foods in each daily box along with plenty of fresh water. On day six, the day after your fast, break the fast gently by consuming small amounts of healthy food, chewing thoroughly, and allowing your body to get used to eating again.

Some find the foods of the ProLon kits overly pricey and restrictive, for example, if you don't like olives, there are no alternatives. For this reason, many people choose a do-it-yourself or DYI option of the FMD on their own, with their own creations. The research on the diet was performed only with the pre-made kits, but many people mimic the fasting mimicking diet by consuming the following nutritional breakdown, based on 1,100 calories for day 1, then 725 calories for days 2-5, which is the same as the ProLon meal boxes. The following macronutrient ratios are used for this copycat FMD strategy:

- Day 1: 30g protein, 56g fat, 117g carbs
- Days 2-5: 16g protein, 35g fat and 85g carbs

The original meal plans are plant-based, and some health professionals believe you will get the best benefits by keeping the DIY options using similar guidelines. The nutritional bar is a healthy nut bar using coconut for fiber. Many find the original bar from ProLong delicious, and so purchase those independently, but others prefer to consume a handful of nuts. Soups can be replaced with similar plant-based, organic soups such as mushroom bisque and split peas. Herbal teas and pitted green olives are easy enough to purchase at most stores, along with seed-based crackers. The glycerol supplement can also be purchased online or in some health food stores.

Just like other diet strategies, planning can make following the FMD easier. Plan the days you will fast, purchase your foods ahead of time and stick with it. Some people claim you can exercise during the fast since you are eating, while others believe you will get more benefits by not exercising. I believe each person should pay attention to their body and exercise as they see fit. Easy walking and stretching can help keep your muscles tuned up while promoting healthy blood and lymphatic flow.

Lastly, the FMD is meant to be performed more than once. The clinical trials showed results when the 5-day fast was followed once each month for three consecutive months. If you decide to try the 5-day plan in the same manner, be sure to stick with a healthy eating plan in between the fasts.

What are the Benefits? The benefits of the FMD are similar to fasting, such as increased stem cell production and weight loss. As mentioned above, these health benefits have been measured with the FMD when the plan was followed once a month for three consecutive months.

- **Fat loss:** In one animal study (with mice), the FMD cycles improved blood glucose and lowered visceral fat. The good news is that after normal, healthy eating was resumed, fat levels did not return to pre-fasting levels. In addition, the study indicated that FMD showed improved signs of liver and muscle regeneration.[16]
- **Improved brain function:** Enhanced cognitive performance was indicated in the same study. Specifically, the regeneration of brain cells in the hippocampus was apparent after three cycles of FMD.[17]
- **Protect from disease:** Another mouse study showed that symptoms of multiple sclerosis (MS) were revered in 20% of animal models, while levels of corticosterone and T cells increased. Both

---

16 White H, Venkatesh B. Clinical review: ketones and brain injury. Crit Care. 2011;15(2):219. Published 2011 Apr 6. doi:10.1186/cc10020

17 Brandhorst S, Choi IY, Wei M, Cheng CW, Sedrakyan S, Navarrete G, Dubeau L, Yap LP, Park R, Vinciguerra M, Di Biase S, Mirzaei H, Mirisola MG, Childress P, Ji L, Groshen S, Penna F, Odetti P, Perin L, Conti PS, Ikeno Y, Kennedy BK, Cohen P, Morgan TE, Dorff TB, Longo VD. A Periodic Diet that Mimics Fasting Promotes Multi-System Regeneration, Enhanced Cognitive Performance, and Healthspan. Cell Metab. 2015 Jul 7;22(1):86-99. doi: 10.1016/j.cmet.2015.05.012. Epub 2015 Jun 18. PMID: 26094889; PMCID: PMC4509734.

of these are important to help reduce internal inflammation and are necessary for a healthy immune system.[18]

- **Improved blood pressure:** In Dr. Longo's original clinical trials, he showed that diastolic blood pressure improvement lasted for at least three months after the three cycles of his FMD program.
- **Convenience:** Convenience is the key motivation for many who purchase pre-packaged meals from the company. This eliminates the need for calculating macronutrients and for finding the right replacement foods. Basically, it takes the thinking out of planning, so you can focus on work or any other responsibilities you may have.

What are the drawbacks? The drawbacks to this meal plan are also similar to fasting: hunger seems to be the biggest complaint. Many people find the foods bland and do not leave them feeling satisfied. By day 5, many develop a distaste for the foods altogether.

Fatigue, headaches, weakness, and sometimes dizziness are the most common drawbacks to regular fasting and FMD is no different since the body is tricked into fasting mode. Some advocates claim that side effects are to a lesser degree because you are eating, but anecdotal evidence shows these side effects can go either way.

More drawbacks that appear to be more specific to FMD include muscle soreness and fatigue, difficulty sleeping, constipation, brain fog, and even sugar cravings. The glycerol drink is meant to help

---

18   Choi IY, Piccio L, Childress P, Bollman B, Ghosh A, Brandhorst S, Suarez J, Michalsen A, Cross AH, Morgan TE, Wei M, Paul F, Bock M, Longo VD. A Diet Mimicking Fasting Promotes Regeneration and Reduces Autoimmunity and Multiple Sclerosis Symptoms. Cell Rep. 2016 Jun 7;15(10):2136-2146. doi: 10.1016/j.celrep.2016.05.009. Epub 2016 May 26. PMID: 27239035; PMCID: PMC4899145.

Whether during Ramadan or for health reasons, studies show short periods of fasting could even improve cognitive function, stimulating faster learning and better memory.

ward off some of these symptoms but also be sure to drink plenty of water during the fast.

Cost is the biggest complaint for this plan. Many believe the price tag does not match the amount of food and nutrition that is supplied in each meal box. But proponents believe the price is worth it as it comes with support and is clinically backed. Nonetheless, if you feel the cost is an issue, the above copycat plan should offer similar benefits.

Who should not do it: The following people should avoid using the FMD:

- Anyone who requires medical oversight for medications
- Women who are pregnant or nursing
- Those under 18 or over 70 years of age
- People who are underweight and/or malnourished
- Those with eating disorders

OMAD or One Meal a Day

OMAD stands for one meal a day and is exactly that – follow the program by eating just one meal a day. It is a form of IF and is also called restricted or time-restricted eating, as you follow the 23/1 rule of fasting, meaning you fast for 23 hours and have a 1-hour feeding window. In its most basic form, there are no food rules or specifications except to fast for 23 hours a day.

What is it? As mentioned, OMAD stands for one meal a day, leaving 23 hours of fasting each day. This is enough time to reap the benefits of fasting such as increased HGH, autophagy, and weight loss. Prominent athletes, like Ronda Rousey and Herschel Walker, practice their own versions of OMAD, and according to food historian Caroline Yeldham, ancient Romans ate only one meal a day and believed it promoted healthy digestion.

Some proponents advocate consuming a healthy meal at your normal dinner time after most of your activity is completed and you are resting for the evening. But if breakfast or lunch are your favorite meals, both are acceptable, as long as you fast for the following 23 hours. And while some people claim to eat anything they want, it is generally accepted by those who advocate or do it to eat healthy foods, since this is your one time of day to eat.

How to: The rules for OMAD are simple: consume one meal a day. Whether your goal is weight loss or improved health, that one meal should provide a well-rounded array of nutrients and around 1,200–1,800 calories, depending on your energetic needs.

Some people prefer to do OMAD every day until they have reached their goals, then may slowly introduce another meal into the day by breaking up the one meal. For example, if you were consuming 1,200 calories in your one meal, you have reached your desired goal, and you're ready to change things up, then you can break up that one meal into two meals of 600 calories each and consume the two meals within eight hours, which will continue the health benefits of IF as you enter the 16/8 phase (16 hours of fasting, 8-hour feeding window).

DIET PLAN

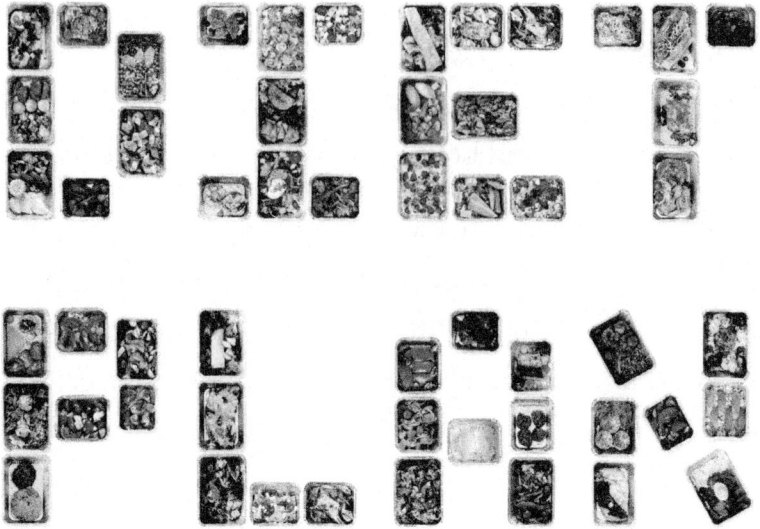

Other proponents advocate incorporating two or three days of OMAD into a weekly schedule while using a different IF plan for the rest of the week. How you choose to incorporate OMAD will depend on your health goals and your lifestyle. Some people may only be able to do OMAD on the weekends, while others only incorporate it Monday through Friday because it is easy to fit into a work schedule.

Putting a well-rounded meal together for your OMAD plan will take some thought. Remember that along with sufficient calories, the body needs healthy fats, protein, and an array of vitamins, minerals, and micronutrients. The following are some examples of OMAD meals:

Breakfast or Early Meal

- 1 cup Greek yogurt
- 2 sausage links
- 2 eggs cooked your way
- 1 ½ cups steamed veggies topped with 1 Tbsp olive oil and 2 Tbsp parmesan cheese

Evening Meal Option 1

- 6 ounces of grilled salmon
- ½ cup of quinoa
- 1 cup of asparagus and 1 cup of carrots, sautéed with 1 Tbsp olive oil and topped with 1 slice of chopped bacon
- 1 small apple
- ½ cup rice pudding with milk and 1 Tbsp almond butter

Evening Meal Option 2

- 1 cooked chicken breast with a creamy mushroom sauce
- 1 cup cauliflower rice with butter
- Roasted Brussels sprouts topped with 1 Tbsp olive oil

The above are just ideas. You can follow your regular meal plan (keto, vegan, paleo, etc.), just make sure that you are getting enough calories in that one meal. By adding more healthy fats, you can easily increase the calories as well.

Planning your meals ahead of time will help you determine approximate calories. Planning for an entire week will help you see the bigger picture to ensure you are con-

> **FAST FACT**
>
> When you take a break from eating, your body is able to focus on other regenerative systems. This allows the body to clean up toxins and regulate the functionality of other organs, including your kidney and liver, which in turn can help clear your skin.

FAST FACT

While fasting, your body uses insulin more efficiently, to take glucose from the blood. Overall, intermittent fasting can lead to a significant reduction in blood sugar levels.

suming a variety of proteins, fat, and vegetables to cover your daily requirements. Also, planning the rest of your day will help keep your mind off food, so schedule activities like walks, visiting friends, going to a movie, reading, or taking up a new hobby.

Implementing herbs like turmeric, ginger, garlic, and Ceylon cinnamon can help stimulate internal detoxification. Also, adding a cup of green tea can stimulate autophagy and boost your metabolism, too. Some prefer to avoid beverages with the meal as it may lessen one's appetite, but you can drink herbal teas throughout the day as long as you add nothing to it. Also, remember to drink plenty of water throughout the day to remain hydrated.

What are the Benefits? OMAD enthusiasts around the world enjoy this type of fast because it is easy. Planning one meal is easier than planning four meals every day, and chances are you will feel satisfied after that one, large meal. In addition, there are fewer dishes to clean, no need to worry about packing a lunch for work if your meal is in the evening, and more time for other activities.

Proponents of OMAD believe this type of eating is instinctively natural for the human body since it is unlikely our ancestors consumed 3 meals plus 2 snacks a day. The time left for fasting allows the body to put energy into the many other functions necessary for healthy living including self-detoxification and healing.

A boost in energy and focus are benefits of OMAD and those who practice it regularly report improved focus and mental clarity. This may be due to ancient survival instincts kicking in while fasting. Research does show that fasting increases levels of norepinephrine, a hormone associated with mental alertness. But fasting also increases the production of dopamine and adrenaline, and the combination can improve mood and brain function. And lastly, the body enters ketosis during the fasting stage of OMAD, and ketones are known to be a superior form of energy for brain cells, resulting in improved mental acuity.

Weight loss is one of the most common side effects of OMAD and may be the result of certain hormonal actions that take place with this type of fasting. By consuming one meal, your body will digest the food from the meal and then rest. When the digestion is at rest, other internal processes can then take place such as autophagy, or internal detoxification. Fasting also improves insulin levels, making weight loss easier, and it helps normalize the hunger hormone called ghrelin. At the same time, the hormone norepinephrine, which was mentioned earlier concerning mental alertness, is also a fat-burning hormone, so not only does your brain go into high power, but so does thermogenesis.

Furthermore, one small study found that people with type 2 diabetes enjoyed improved blood glucose levels when fasting 18 to 20 hours a day.[19] OMAD can certainly help one achieve this.

19   Arnason TG, Bowen MW, Mansell KD. Effects of intermittent fasting on health markers in those with type 2 diabetes: A pilot study. *World J Diabetes.* 2017;8(4):154-164. doi:10.4239/wjd.v8.i4.154

Contrary to popular thinking, fasting helps preserve muscle mass and with the right meals, OMAD can even help you build muscle. That's because when fasting, the body converts defective proteins as a fuel supply, instead of muscle protein. Also, during autophagy, the body releases hormones like somatropin, which preserves muscles. And lastly, fasting stimulates HGH, which is a known stimulant for muscle growth. So, when you incorporate OMAD, be sure to include high-quality protein with your meal along with other highly nutritious foods to get the most benefits during the fasting stage. Weight training will help you build more muscle, which becomes more and more important as we get older.

What are the drawbacks? One of the biggest drawbacks to OMAD is the promotion of being able to eat what you want. Fasting for 23 hours will only cause illness and lethargy if your one meal consists of junk foods or highly processed foods that are often devoid of nutrition. In fact, many junk foods not only lack nutrition, but they leech what precious reserves you have to help your body break them down, leaving you nutritionally depleted.

OMAD may require more discipline for some, as fasting for 23 hours can be a challenge. If you choose dinner or breakfast as your one meal and you work at a job, you will have to find other things to do with your lunch break, such as run errands, read, or take a walk.

Other drawbacks of OMAD are similar to other fasting plans such as fatigue, headache, bad breath, brain fog, and physical weakness. While this seems contrary to some of the benefits, everybody will have periods of feeling great and then not so great, depending upon the internal processes that are taking place. For example, autophagy might stimulate the release of certain toxins that can make you feel bad as they dislodge.

One of the reasons people do OMAD is to avoid the common drawbacks of fasting while taking advantage of the benefits. Again, consuming a healthy meal and staying hydrated can help control some symptoms. However, if your health needs improving, it might take some time for your body to get used to fasting straight for 23 hours. If you have trouble doing the full 23 hours, try drinking broth or water with a little lemon juice in it.

Who should not do it: Because of the strictness of OMAD, those under 18 years of age should avoid this fast. At the same time, elderly people and people who are underweight, pregnant, or nursing should also not fast.

People with health conditions or medications should talk to their doctor before embarking on any fast. With that being said, OMAD might be the right kind of fast to help you get your health in check, so talk to your doctor and if you get the go-ahead, ask them to help monitor your health. You both might be pleasantly surprised with the results!

The Warrior Diet

Sometimes referred to as the cousin of the OMAD fast, the Warrior Diet is another form of IF, or intermittent fasting, and may also be called the 20:4 fasting cycle. This form of IF, however, was developed by a former member of the Israeli Special Forces, Ori Hofmekler. He admits there is no scientific data or research to back up his particular fasting plan, however, many followers believe it does work and shares the benefits of other forms of IF.

What is it? The Warrior Diet is a diet plan in which you undereat for 20 hours of the day and then overeat for four hours, preferably in the evening. While most forms of IF encourage eating anything you desire on feeding days, Mr. Hofmekler promotes eating a clean diet of unprocessed foods, dairy, protein, and plenty of fresh vegetables and fruits. He claims this eating pattern is based on ancient warriors who fasted during the long training or fighting days and then feasted at night.

How to: This plan is divided into three phases that each last for one week. You should consume the type of food explained in each phase for a total of approximately 2,000 calories a day. Follow each week in order, then at the end of the initial three weeks, you can either repeat the phases again or simply follow a 20/4 IF cycle in which you eat within a four-hour window and then fast for 20 hours until your next 4-hour feeding window. The phases are as follows:

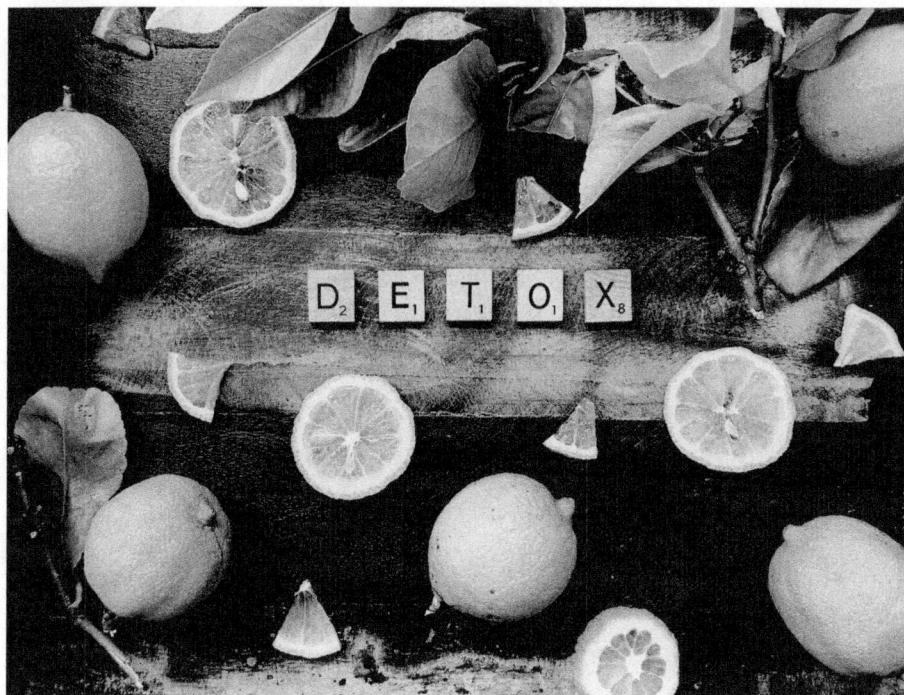

Phase I Detox

Fast 20 hours: "Undereat" for 20 hours, beginning from the time you get out of bed (of course, the 6 to 8 hours you sleep you will not eat, and it does count as part of the 20 hours fasting period). To begin, take note of the time you consumed your last meal before you begin the Warrior Diet. If you ate at 8:00 pm, that is your last meal. Your next full meal cannot take place until 4 pm the next afternoon.

After you rise the next morning, you will consume only: black tea or coffee, small portions of vegetables, fruits, plain yogurt, hard-boiled eggs, cottage cheese, and vegetable juice (such as celery). Do not consume meat, poultry, or fish. While no calorie restrictions are followed, it is generally understood to just eat small portions of food, choosing from the above list. Consume only small portions or small servings to curb hunger pangs, but do not eat an entire meal until 4:00 pm (based on the last meal at 8:00 pm the previous evening).

Feast 4 hours: Dinner time is when the feeding window begins, and the time to "overeat." Begin with a serving of healthy food and wait 20 minutes. If you are still hungry, eat another small meal and wait 20 minutes. Repeat this pattern, eating as often as you need to for a total of four hours.

Dinner meal choices include:

Begin each feeding window with a salad with olive oil and vinegar dressing. After 20 minutes, choose from the following meals (you can choose more than one to make a complete meal):

- Bowl of steamed vegetables
- 1 cup of lentils, edamame, black beans or kidney beans
- 1 cup of barley, quinoa or brown rice
- Hummus
- One ounce of kefir, goat cheese, yogurt, feta cheese, or ricotta cheese
- 2 poached eggs

Stop eating all candies, desserts, bread, or sugary foods. Do not add sugar or sweetener to beverages and drink plenty of water throughout the day.

Phase 2 High Fat

Fast 20 hours: Undereat for 20 hours with clear broths, vegetable juice, raw fruits and/or vegetables, cottage cheese, or yogurt.

Feast 4 hours: When the 20 hours are up, begin your four-hour feeding window with a salad using olive oil and vinegar as dressing. Wait 20 minutes and then eat a meal of lean animal protein and steamed vegetables. After 20 minutes or when you are hungry again (within the four hours), eat a handful of soaked nuts. Do not consume grains or starches during this phase.

Phase 3 Concluding Fat Loss

During this phase, you must cycle between high-carb meals and high-protein meals. The following is the pattern:

- 1-2 days of high carbs
- 1-2 days of low carbs / high protein
- Repeat the above until the week is complete.

Follow the pattern of eating as in phase 2 of 20 hours of undereating and 4 hours of overeating. BUT – add the high carbs foods during the four-hour feeding or overeating window. The carb selection is as follows:

- Oats
- Corn
- Sweet potatoes
- Peas

> **FAST FACT**
>
> Intermittent fasting can decrease blood pressure, increase insulin sensitivity, and increase heart rate variability, all of which decrease the risk of developing cardiovascular diseases and strokes.

- Pumpkin
- Quinoa
- Pasta
- Whole grain bread
- Barley
- Rice

The trick to this plan is to eat scant meals during the fasting part, and during the overeating period consume small, healthy meals with 20 minutes in between. This 20-minute window helps you to avoid overeating, which can lead to discomfort and digestive issues.

The creator of this plan also recommends including nutritional supplements that you feel are needed, such as a multivitamin and mineral supplement. Also, exercise most days of the week, with at least two days of strength training.

What are the benefits? The Warrior Diet is a form of intermittent fasting that is backed by clinical evidence. The 20/4 fasting plan is included in some studies that show it does result in weight loss and lowered risk for cardiovascular disease. (Stote et al., 2007) Weight loss can improve blood pressure, which lowers the risk of other chronic diseases as well.

Additionally, fasting for 18-20 hours a day also improves post-meal blood sugar levels, which can ultimately reduce cravings, especially if you stick with healthy eating during feeding windows. Sticking with the actual food plan instead of the general theory of eating any meal you desire will provide greater benefits.

Lastly, even if you cheat during feeding windows, the fasting period will help your digestion rest and reset. The result is that you will still see benefits, like an improvement in overall blood sugar and insulin levels.

Because you consume calories throughout the day, this program provides enough energy so you can still exercise. Some people feel they have more energy while on this fasting plan, and so can lose even more weight.

What are the drawbacks? Hunger is the biggest drawback of the Warrior Diet. This may be because extended fasts often lead to lesser hunger while the meals consumed with this program may trigger increased hunger for some people. Most people do not use this diet as a way of life, but to lead into another improved lifestyle diet plan or to lose weight.

This type of IF is not easy and may take time for your body to adjust. Some people may experience the same side effects as extended fasting including fatigue, brain fog, nausea, and less commonly, hormonal disruptions (depending on the lifestyle leading into the fast). The side effects often resolve as the body becomes accustomed to this way of eating. Hormonal disruptions might be experienced by those with hormonal issues or those taking medications.

Who should not do it: People on medications or with health issues should either avoid this fast or consult their doctor before beginning this type of fast. People with eating disorders or who have an unhealthy relationship with food should not do this fast, as experts believe it can lead to obsessive thoughts about food. Those who are

FAST FACT

Fat burning typically begins after approximately 12 hours of fasting and escalates between 16 and 24 hours of fasting.

under 18 and people who are underweight, pregnant, or nursing should not follow this fast.

ADF or Alternate Day Fasting

Alternate day fasting is a way to lose weight and take advantage of fasting, but by restricting your food intake only half the time. In other words, you fast on one day followed by a day of eating without calorie restrictions. Fasting days allow a small intake of calories of up to 25% of your normal caloric intake and with some recommendations instructing you to consume no more than 500 calories on fasting days.

ADF is commonly described as alternating days of fasting with days of no calorie restrictions and no food guidelines. However, as with any type of diet, you will not achieve your goals very quickly if you fill up on junk food during the times that you can eat. In fact, some studies that show ADF had a similar impact on weight loss as calorie restriction did not consider the diet. However other studies showed ADF with sensible meals on non-fasting days resulted in weight loss as well as the myriad of other benefits associated with intermittent fasting (IF), therefore if you try this, do your best to eat well when you are not fasting.

What is it? Alternate-day fasting is a form of IF. In this version, you fast every other day or on alternate days. Some who follow ADF may abstain from food altogether on fasting days, drinking only water and herbal teas, while another may consume 500 calories on their fasting days. The point is to either fast or trick the body into fasting mode on a regular basis.

ADF may sometimes be referred to as Eat-Stop-Eat after a popular fasting program developed by author Brad Pilon, who advocated two 24-hour fasts each week with normal, healthy eating during the other days. It was meant to make healthy eating easier for anyone without the need for special tools, counting calories or macronutrients, and still providing benefits like weight loss and increased productivity.

How to: A typical week plan would be to fast on Monday, Wednesday, Friday, and Sunday and continue fasting the following week on Tuesday, Thursday and Saturday. The result is that you are fasting three days one week and four days the following week, which will continue to alternate as long as you follow the same protocol.

It is encouraged to eat as you normally would during non-fasting days. However, eating junk foods and highly processed foods can leave you feeling sick while consuming too many carbs may trigger cravings that follow you into the next day. I believe it's best to proceed with as many healthy and whole foods as possible.

On fasting days, consume only water, black coffee, and tea with nothing added. Each day that you don't fast, eat healthy meals at normal times. The bottom line is to simply fast every other day, so choose the days to fast that are easiest to fit into your schedule for at least the first couple of weeks.

Some people choose to follow a modified fast, in which they consume 500 calories instead of zero calories. Studies that have shown the benefits of ADF are most often performed with modified fasting because it is considered more sustainable. Yet studies that showed alternate day fasting with zero calories on fasting days resulted in increased fat oxidation and lower insulin levels in non-obese participants.[20]

Choosing a zero-calorie fast or modified fast depends upon your health and lifestyle. Consuming any food on fasting days triggers some people to eat more meals, so it may be more difficult for some. However, adding a 500-calorie meal to a fasting day helps those with high activity levels stick with ADF more easily.

What are the Benefits? Many people find ADF easier to follow than calorie restriction. This may be because it is encouraged to eat what you want on feeding days and to consume 500 to 600 calories on fasting days. Overall, many find the flexibility easy as they can look forward to a full meal after just one day of fasting. At the same time, some people feel fasting every other day strengthens their willpower.

---

20   Heilbronn LK, Smith SR, Martin CK, Anton SD, Ravussin E. Alternate-day fasting in nonobese subjects: effects on body weight, body composition, and energy metabolism. Am J Clin Nutr. 2005 Jan;81(1):69-73. doi: 10.1093/ajcn/81.1.69. PMID: 15640462.

Weight loss was found to be a benefit that anyone can enjoy whether following a strict fast or a modified fast with ADF. Along with weight loss, most people can experience reduced insulin levels and lowered risk factors for type 2 diabetes when following ADF, and the benefits will last as long as one continues to eat healthily.

Furthermore, ADF can improve heart health for individuals who are overweight or obese. That's because risk factors like blood pressure, bad cholesterol (LDL), waist circumference, and blood triglycerides all decrease. In addition, ADF promotes longevity as it reduces oxidative damage to our cells.[21]

As mentioned with other types of fasting, ADF stimulates autophagy, which improves health as your body naturally eliminates used-up and damaged cells, thus reducing the risk of chronic disease and certain cancers.

Benefits are found with ADF in every study, regardless of the participants being of normal weight or obese and whether they were strict in fasting or followed a modified fast. Interestingly, none of the studies kept track of the actual foods that were consumed during the trials. We can assume then that ADF would provide even more benefits if very healthy eating were followed at mealtimes!

In fact, one study conducted by Krista Varady, Ph.D., divided participants into a high-fat group that obtained 45% of their calories from fat and another group that obtained 25% of their calories from fat. The high-fat group lost 17 pounds over eight weeks while

21   Harvie MN, Pegington M, Mattson MP, et al. The effects of intermittent or continuous energy restriction on weight loss and metabolic disease risk markers: a randomized trial in young overweight women. Int J Obes (Lond). 2011;35(5):714-727. doi:10.1038/ijo.2010.171

the lower-fat group lost an average of 12 to 13 pounds. This was attributed to the fact that the high-fat group felt more satiated and therefore cheated less than the low-fat group.[22]

An often-overlooked benefit of fasting is increased productivity. While some researchers may contribute this to improved cognitive skills, others believe it is because one can get more things done on fasting days when not worrying about preparing and cleaning up after meals. Since the fast is only one day, many people do not experience a drop in energy until towards the end of the day, and the lack of energy indicates one should rest, anyway.

What are the drawbacks? The most observed drawback to ADF was a 10% to 40% dropout rate that seemed to pan across all studies. However, for those who stick with it, it is interesting that eating days resulted in participants consuming no more than 110% of their normal calories, which is still a considerable deficit.[23]

Hunger is another issue with ADF, as some people find it difficult to begin a new fast every day. When fasting for longer periods, the often-euphoric feeling and high energy that comes with longer fasts make them easier to stick to, whereas a 24-hour fast (or 36 if you count sleeping) may not offer those physical and mental sensations.

Who should not do it: People who have eating disorders should not try ADF, as well as people who are underweight or pregnant/nursing. If you have any health issues or take medications, ADF may

---

22 Wisby, G. (2013, February 5). Krista Varady weighs in on how to drop pounds. Retrieved May 05, 2021, from https://today.uic.edu/krista-varady-weighs-in-on-how-to-drop-pounds-fast

23 Trepanowski JF, Kroeger CM, Barnosky A, et al. Effect of Alternate-Day Fasting on Weight Loss, Weight Maintenance, and Cardioprotection Among Metabolically Healthy Obese Adults: A Randomized Clinical Trial. JAMA Intern Med. 2017;177(7):930-938. doi:10.1001/jamainternmed.2017.0936

be an option, but you should always check with your doctor before beginning any type of fast.

5:2 Diet

The 5:2 fast is another form of IF, and I included it here because you may come across it in other fasting literature as a separate type of fast. It is a fast in its own right, as it was created or popularized by the previously mentioned journalist and fasting advocate and expert, Michael Mosley.

What is it? This type of IF is popular for weight loss and includes regular full fasting each week. The plan also promotes consuming 500 to 600 calories on fasting days. Many people find it easy to follow as it follows the typical mantra of, *it's not what you eat, but the time you eat it.*

How to: This plan is fairly straightforward in that you eat "normally" for five days each week. The other two days should include enough food to make up about 25% of your normal, daily calories, so as in other fasts, about 500 calories for women and 600 for men.

Also, as with other plans, the "normal" eating plan should not include junk foods, highly processed foods, or excessive sweets, desserts, and high-sugar beverages. You should consume your normal number of calories from healthy, preferably unprocessed foods that include wholesome proteins, vegetables, healthy fats, some fruits, and very low carbs for best results.

Because this fast includes five eating days, planning will bring greater success. Plan the days you will eat and the days you will fast. Plan your meals ahead of time, including the small meals or snacks you will eat on fasting days. Write out your daily meal plans and post them where you can see them. Then purchase your food ahead of time so you are not swayed. Unless you have incredible willpower, avoid eating at restaurants for a while and avoid carbs in order to avoid cravings. The more you plan and stick with it, the greater success you will have.

During normal eating days, try to follow your regular pattern of eating. On fasting days, break up your calories into two or three small meals. Since the caloric allotment is small, focus on making your calories count by consuming highly nutritious foods that will help you reach your goals. Some meal examples include:

• Unsweetened yogurt with berries
• 2 boiled or poached eggs
• A mixture of steamed vegetables with a little butter, ghee, or coconut oil
• Grilled lean meat or fish with a small salad

What are the Benefits? This type of diet was popularized as an effective way to lose weight. Many people find it easier to stick with since there are only two fasting days with normal calorie consumption on the other days. Interestingly, most people who follow this type of fast did not eat to make up for calories on non-fasting days.

This fast is effective for weight loss and promotes the loss of abdominal fat, which in turn lowers your risk for many chronic diseases. In fact, it was shown to lead to an average of 3 to 8% of weight loss over 3-24 weeks, with some losing 4-7% of their belly fat.[24] The results are more apparent when combined with strength training twice each week or some form of cardio exercise four times each week.

The 5:2 way of IF was used in a clinical trial at the Family History (Genetics) Clinic at the Genesis Prevention Centre, University Hospital of South Manchester. The participants were women ages 20 to 69 years. The participants were instructed to consume 25% of their caloric intake on two consecutive days of each week. During non-fasting days, they were instructed to consume a Mediterranean type of diet that included lean proteins, dairy, vegetables, and low-carbohydrate fruits. Compared to the control group, the participants of the IF groups lost more body fat and saw improved insulin levels. They also noted lower markers for cardiovascular disease and higher ketones in their blood, which is believed to protect against metabolic and age-related diseases.[25]

What are the drawbacks? There are published studies that show the 5:2 fast did not show significantly more benefits than calorie-restricted diets, however, it must be noted that during these studies, participants were instructed to eat their normal diet. Because there was no record of the diets of the participants, they could have been consuming pizza and burgers on their feeding days. On the other hand, the research mentioned above found 5:2 to be very successful

---

24 Adrienne R. Barnosky, Kristin K. Hoddy, Terry G. Unterman, Krista A. Varady, Intermittent fasting vs daily calorie restriction for type 2 diabetes prevention: a review of human findings, Translational Research, Volume 164, Issue 4, 2014, Pages 302-311, ISSN 1931-5244, https://doi.org/10.1016/j.trsl.2014.05.013.

25 Harvie M, Wright C, Pegington M, et al. The effect of intermittent energy and carbohydrate restriction v. daily energy restriction on weight loss and metabolic disease risk markers in overweight women. Br J Nutr. 2013;110(8):1534-1547. doi:10.1017/S0007114513000792

when participants were instructed to consume a healthy diet; in this case the Mediterranean diet. This is yet more proof that, no matter what type of IF you try, a healthy diet is still imperative for the best results.

Other drawbacks of this type of fasting are similar to other fasting programs. The side effects may include nausea, hunger, light-headedness, or fatigue. This often resolves on its own as the body becomes used to limited calories. Side effects are highly individual, but seem to be less with those who are used to fasting or for those with fewer health conditions.

Hunger is the most commonly reported side effect of the 5:2 fast, as with most forms of IF. This is very common for those who have never fasted for an entire day before. However, many people find it more tolerable after the first two fasting days, while some simply feel more energized and lighter during the fasting days.

Who should not do it: People who are underweight and under 18 should not embark on this type of fast. It's also not suitable for pregnant or nursing mothers. Also, those with eating disorders should avoid most forms of IF, as it may trigger binge eating. Lastly, anyone taking medications or with medical conditions should either avoid this fast or talk to their doctor to see if they are healthy enough to fast and if it would be beneficial for them.

4:3 Diet

The 4:3 diet is another form of IF, and I included it here because you may come across it in other fasting literature as a separate type of fast.

What is it? The 4:3 diet is sometimes called alternate-day fasting (ADF). The numbers represent four days a week in which you consume regular meals, while the three is the number of days you fast. However, in this particular fast, the fasting days should be modified by consuming an average of 500 calories each fasting day.

How to: Because this is another form of IF in which it is encouraged to not change your diet, preparation does not need to be as intense as a zero-calorie prolonged fast of three days or longer. Because 4:3 includes three fasting days, many people find they have more self-control on feeding days and use this time to ease into a healthier lifestyle with an improved diet.

To incorporate the 4:3 fast, plan which days you will fast and which days you will eat. The fasting days should not be consecutive, and you can include 500 calories (600 for men). The calories can be consumed in one meal or broken down into 2-3 small meals. Be sure to drink plenty of water and, of course, you can drink black coffee and tea.

Fasting day meals should include fresh vegetables and fruits with high-quality protein. Some proponents include oatmeal or other grains; however, this may trigger cravings in some people. It is best to play around with your meals to see how your body responds and what works best for you. Please note that the studies below included only participants who fasted with zero calories, however, some experts claim that consuming 500 calories for women and 600 for men provides the same benefits.

On your normal, or feeding days, it is encouraged to eat as you want so you feel satisfied. However, many people will find if they eat foods that are not healthy, such as heavy, fried foods, or highly processed foods, they may feel nauseous or tired. It is best to consume healthy fats and protein and low carbohydrates for the best results.

What are the Benefits? The benefits of the 4:3 fasting program have clinical studies that show its effectiveness. Fasting in this fashion has been shown to be beneficial and safe for extended periods of six months or longer for healthy adults.

In at least one study, participants who were considered obese enjoyed weight loss on 4:3 and most found it easier to stick with than calorie-restricted diets. This may be because on the days you eat, there are no restrictions, so you don't feel deprived. At the same time, long-term calorie restriction can lead to muscle and bone loss whereas alternate-day fasting has been shown not to cause such issues.

This type of fasting has resulted in a reduction of overall body mass, as well as a reduction in abdominal fat. A review of ADF studies found that blood levels of polyunsaturated fatty acids, or PUFAs improved, which points to a lowered risk of numerous, chronic diseases like heart disease and diabetes mellitus. Also, ADF led to a depletion of methionine, which is an amino acid that is associated with aging. These benefits were compiled into a report that determined ADF improves fat-to-lean bodyweight ratio with an average of 4.5% of body weight reduction in four weeks, along with the above longevity benefits. (Stekovic et al., 2019)

Other benefits of the 4:3 fast include reduced insulin resistance, better tolerance to allergies, less risk for asthma attacks, and improved heart arrhythmias. These benefits were found when a study group was compared to a group of participants that ate normally. (Johnson et al., 2016)

What are the drawbacks? While this fasting pattern has proven safe for most people, the main drawback is the dropout rate. It is reported that the hunger remains on fasting days, even after following the program for over a month. On the other hand, some who have issues with hunger claim that their discipline strengthens when they stick with the 4:3.

Who should not do it: Intermittent fasting like the 4:3 diet should not be done by people who are malnourished or underweight, as it could exacerbate the issue. People who are under 18 and women who are pregnant or nursing should also not follow this program.

If you are under any type of medical treatment or taking medications, always check with your doctor or healthcare provider about fasting to ensure it is a safe practice for your level of health.

Dry Fasting

This fast is saved for last as it is the most extreme form of fasting and is best for only seasoned or experienced fasters who are in good health. It is commonly used for religious purposes, but also offers some very real benefits. Dry fasting is reportedly the fact that Moses, Ezra, and even Jesus Christ of the Bible used. Even Jonah (of

Jonah and the whale fame) supposedly embarked on a dry fast for three days.

Dry fasting is recorded in Russian literature for intense healing. Doctors and practitioners in Russia not only recommend it to their patients but also suggest fasting in the fresh air of the mountains and sleeping next to a stream or running water.

What is it? Dry fasting is done by abstaining from all food and drinks, even water. Some experts claim that one day of this type of fasting is equivalent to three days of fasting with water. That makes this type of fast more efficient as the body can perform more healing or detox functions in a shorter time.

There are two types of dry fasting: soft dry fast and hard dry fast. Both involve abstaining from food and water, however, a soft dry fast allows you to come into contact with water such as during teeth brushing or showering. A hard dry fast, on the other hand, is done by total abstinence from contact with water, both inside and outside of your body.

Advocates of dry fasting believe it is one of the most convenient ways to fast. Simply practice fasting on any days that are convenient to you, whether it's one day per week or once each month. And most certainly do not jump into dry fasting, as it can be dangerous if your body is not prepared.

How to: While this form of fasting is simple, you just abstain from all food and drinks, including water, there are some guidelines to make your fast productive. Dry fasting is not right for everyone and if you are not a seasoned faster, please start with IF, water fasting, and then slowly you can build up to a short dry fast.

Instead of jumping right into dry fasting, try incorporating it into an intermittent fast, such as a 16/8 plan. Once the eight hours of your eating window is complete, it is time for 16 hours of fasting. Keep in mind that we are already dry fasting every night for 7-8 hours. To extend your dry fast time, plan what time you will abstain from even water or other beverages to extend your "natural" dry fast period until you can do a full 16 hours. Experiment with both soft and hard dry fasting to see how you feel. Once you complete that, you will have a feel for how your body responds to the dry fast.

Once you have tested the waters by dry fasting during a form of IF, you might wish to try a full 24 hours of soft dry fasting. During this time, you can wash your hands, brush your teeth, and shower as usual. After you are able to do this, try a full day of hard dry fasting.

Dr. Sergei Filonov, a Russian medical doctor, uses dry fasting in his practice and recommends trying what he calls cascade fasting. In this method, you dry fast for 1 day, then eat for 1 day, dry fast for 2 days consecutively then eat for 2 days consecutively, and continue in this manner until you reach 5 consecutive days of dry fasting alternated with 5 consecutive days of eating. The result is that you literally dry fast for half the month. He finds this method helps the body adjust more easily while reducing what he calls the "healing crisis," which is the time your body is going through detoxification and shedding high amounts of toxins to be eliminated. Please keep in mind that this is only done with Dr. Filonov's supervision! Do not do this at home!

No matter how you choose to incorporate dry fasting, take it easy and relax as much as possible during this time. Avoid exercise and getting overheated or sweating. Your body heals itself during rest, so allow it this time. Please note that there will be an upcoming section on preparing for any fast. Read that over before embarking on the dry fast, which can be intense to some.

Once your dry fast is complete, spend time easing out of it by slowly sipping water and holding it in your mouth for a few seconds before you swallow it. After sipping water for two hours, drink more water and slowly add diluted juice. You can add some vegetable or bone broth a couple of hours later. Wait another couple of hours and then you should be ready for a light meal.

Aside from slowly allowing your body to begin consuming liquid and food again, be careful with exercise. If you stopped exercising, begin with general stretching or yoga to begin blood circulation and take it from there. A general rule of dry fasting is that you should allow your body to recover for a full day for each day of dry fasting.

What are the Benefits? When dry fasting, the body is deprived of external forms of energy, therefore it will instead use internal sources of energy. Contrary to what seems logical, abstaining from water forces your body to use fat as a form of metabolic water! In fact, for every 100 grams of fat, your body can manufacture about 110 grams of water![26] The result is thermogenesis as your body melts fat to use as a source of fluids.

---

26 MELLANBY, K. Metabolic Water and Desiccation. Nature 150, 21 (1942). https://doi.org/10.1038/150021a0

Because of the thermogenesis, advocates of dry fasting claim fasters will lose less muscle and more fat. The fasting time is less, which leaves less chance for muscle loss, but fat utilization is increased since it quickly becomes a form of energy.

Autophagy is a benefit of most forms of fasting, but when it comes to dry fasting the effects are more impressive. The destruction of used-up and toxic cells within the body normally takes place as the body dislodges them and removes them, or in some cases destroys the cells and then moves them out. However, it seems that during dry fasting, the body burns toxic cells where they are, instead of excreting them, as they are the first to be used for energy. In other words, the toxic cells do not have to travel through the body to be removed. It is believed this is the reason why those who dry fast do not experience foul breath and odor during their fasts, which commonly accompanies traditional water fasting.

Cell regeneration seems to take place during dry fasting, which means it could improve immune function and have anti-aging properties. Cell regeneration is a natural result of autophagy, as the body must replenish the spent cells that have been either destroyed or removed. This would also help explain some of the following benefits.

In a review of studies on Ramadan fasting, which is dry fasting by abstaining from all food and beverages, including water, from sundown to sunup. It is found that dry fasting protects the brain and even improves brain function by increasing levels of **BDNF**, a brain protein that promotes the survival and growth of brain cells.[27]

Similar studies also found that dry fasting quickly reduced internal inflammation, a condition linked to numerous chronic diseases, balanced blood cholesterols, lowered blood pressure, and reduced the risk for coronary disease and diabetes. It also improved bone health by increasing the parathyroid hormone (**PTH**) which in turn led to improved bone resorption, formation, and even an increase in bone calcium.[28]

What are the drawbacks? The drawback is that the body will need more time to heal after a dry fast, or health complications might arise, as mentioned above. If you try this method of fasting, follow the guidelines about how to come out of this type of fast for safety reasons. If you have any doubts, concerns, or questions, talk to your doctor or employ the assistance of a health practitioner to monitor you during your fast.

Moreover, hunger and thirst are the other obvious drawbacks to dry fasting. This is a serious fast that comes with real benefits. Be sure to ease into the fast correctly, as this may help eliminate some of the hunger. Also, the "practice" or short-term dry fasting periods will help your body become accustomed to dry fasting and you should feel better, mentally, about abstaining from water. Some people

27   Longo VD, Mattson MP. Fasting: molecular mechanisms and clinical applications. Cell Metab. 2014;19(2):181-192. doi:10.1016/j.cmet.2013.12.008

28   Bahijri SM, Ajabnoor GM, Borai A, Al-Aama JY, Chrousos GP. Effect of Ramadan fasting in Saudi Arabia on serum bone profile and immunoglobulins. Ther Adv Endocrinol Metab. 2015;6(5):223-232. doi:10.1177/2042018815594527

even find this part more palatable because their empty stomachs do not have to fill up on water.

The side effects of dry fasting are similar to other forms of fasting but may feel more intense. These include hunger, nausea, fatigue, and sometimes headaches. Note, in short-term dry fasting, such as from sundown to sunup, these side effects are less and often not seen by those who are experienced in fasting. If you have been accustomed to consuming sugar, caffeine, or even processed foods, you may feel more side effects as your body detoxifies itself from those substances.

Who should not do it: There are certain situations in which it is not recommended to use dry fasting, such as:

- Those with malignant tumors
- Anyone with blood conditions
- Those with tuberculosis, hyperthyroidism, and other endocrine diseases
- People with cirrhosis of the liver
- Anyone with a heart arrhythmia
- Those who are underweight
- Pregnant or nursing mothers
- Anyone under 18 years of age

As with any fast or extreme diet change, if you have a medical condition or take any type of medication, consult with your doctor to ensure you are healthy enough to dry fast.

CHAPTER 4

The Benefits of Fasting

T HERE ARE LITERALLY HUNDREDS OF STUDIES THAT PROVE THE benefits of fasting are real for humans. Researchers continuously trace the benefits back to our ancestors and our current built-in ability to feast and fast. It appears we are made to survive for long periods of no food consumption, and not only are we made for it, but it makes us stronger! The surprising results of the numerous studies are not simply that the body can survive, but that we thrive when intermittent fasting (IF) is used periodically throughout our lives.

It seems that fasting not only sets a survival instinct in motion, but the human organism overcomes the challenge of starvation by restoring homeostasis. Then, miraculously, cells throughout the entire body engage in a coordinated effort of rebuilding, which leads to the increased expression of DNA repair, autophagy, a reduction of internal inflammation, protein quality control, and improved antioxidant responses along with other strengthened immune responses.

Furthermore, randomized, controlled clinical trials on various animal species demonstrate that a variety of forms of IF counteract disease processes, enhance mitochondrial health, promote cell and DNA repair, and promote stem cell regeneration. All research, whether human or animal, is pointing to the fact that IF is a tool that many people can use to prevent and even manage major chronic diseases, including diseases associated with aging.

Previously, I covered many different styles and plans of IF along with their unique benefits. I tried to point out the benefits that are prominent in each one, however, they actually cross over and seem to encompass all forms of IF. In this section, I will break down the benefits and attempt to explain why they take place and in whom.

Keep in mind that any benefits you receive or don't receive directly coincide with your level of health and your diet during non-fasting days. You cannot expect to get results by fasting three days a week and then filling up on pizza or fast food during normal eating days.

Weight Loss

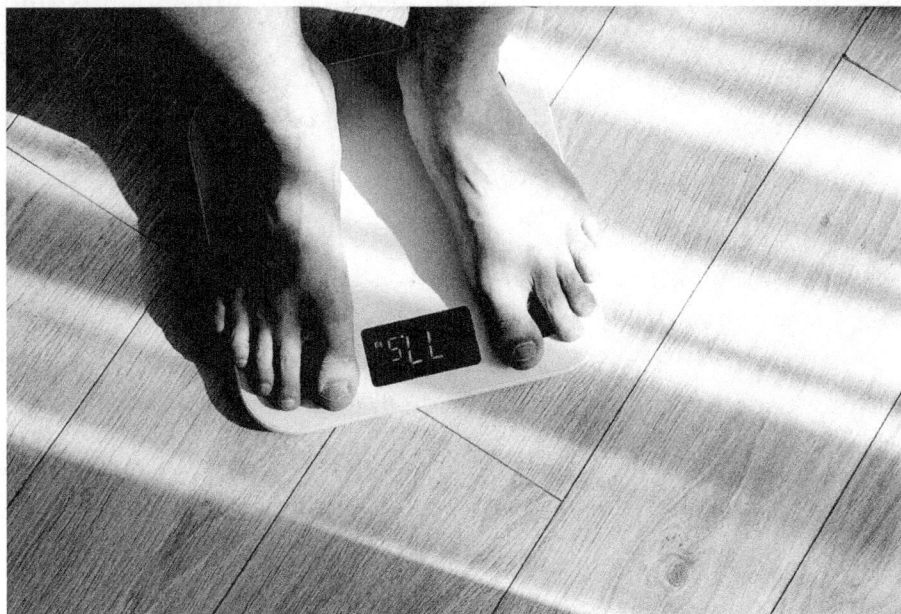

Weight loss is the main reason why people choose to fast. If done correctly, it can be easier than typical dieting since there are no calories to count and no macronutrients to calculate. Just drink water, coffee, and tea or snack on healthy foods that will amount to under 500 calories to reach the fasting goal. Whether you choose water fasting, dry fasting or IF, you will consume fewer calories in a month than your normal diet, without all the fuss, as long as you don't make up for the calories on the other days. But consuming fewer calories is not the only reason fasting leads to weight loss.

When we fast, our digestion has time to rest and reset. Our bodies have miraculous healing abilities that kick in when we don't use energy for digestion, and the energy includes healing the digestive tract by resetting the microbiome. It may do this through the natural process of autophagy while some experts believe it is accomplished by simply resting. No matter the reason, it is well known that the healthier our weight is, the healthier our digestion is, and vice versa.

There are other factors along with fewer calories that contribute to weight loss, such as fasting promotes ketosis, where your body burns fat for fuel instead of carbohydrates. In fact, if you have ever had problems going into ketosis on a low-carb diet, fasting can help you move easily into that state, and burn more fat.

Fasting decreases insulin levels, and when insulin decreases, lipolysis (the fat-burning process) increases. While fasting, your body increases the production of epinephrine and norepinephrine, which are catecholamines that activate lipase to burn more fat. And lastly, fasting increases growth hormone, which naturally boosts metabolism. As you can see, fasting promotes weight loss through numerous pathways!

Anti-Aging

Anti-Aging is an exciting benefit of fasting. As studies pointed out in the previous chapter, fasting improves blood insulin levels, which in turn improves metabolism by causing the body to burn more fat. This hormonal change is also linked to longevity and of course, lowers the risk for diabetes and other chronic or age-related diseases.

Fasting also promotes autophagy, or the process through which the body removes spent cells. Some of these cells may be free radicals, which damage cells and often lead to premature aging. Also, we know that fasting causes the body to use fats as a source of energy, however, that is not the only source. Fasting improves levels of purines and pyrimidines, which are nitrogen bases that hold DNA strands together. But these elements also boost antioxidant production, which fights free radicals. Since free radicals are one factor of premature aging, removing these can only boost longevity.

Furthermore, protecting brain health is another important aspect of anti-aging, and as we have previously seen, fasting improves brain health. To recap, fasting increases ketones levels, which are then used for energy, and ketones are a superior source of energy for the brain. In addition, the process of autophagy helps remove spent or damaged cells, and this includes the brain, thus further protecting it from damage that often comes with age.

Autophagy

Autophagy is the natural process described above in which the body undergoes natural detoxification and destroys or removes cells that are damaged, old or no longer useful. This process is stimulated through fasting, and picks up momentum as fasting continues. When people experience a healing crisis or side effects, it may very well be due to the fact that the old and diseased cells are being dislodged and removed from the body.

One incredible talent of the body is the ability to regenerate cells. When autophagy kicks in, the body destroys or removes harmful cells and then goes into survival mode to regenerate new cells that replace the old, damaged ones. These new cells are fresh, healthy, full of life, and can be created throughout the body including the heart, brain, liver, muscles, and skin. Fresh, healthy cells function more efficiently and fully than the old ones, so in a sense, this is the body self-healing itself.

Autophagy "shapes" mitochondria through a process called selective degradation, which simply means parts of the mitochondria that no longer function properly or at full capacity are broken down to make room to rebuild and promote cell survival. Healthy mitochondria are an important factor in energy levels. The same process also takes place within our DNA strands, allowing it to repair and rebuild which protects our genes, among other things.

Stem Cells

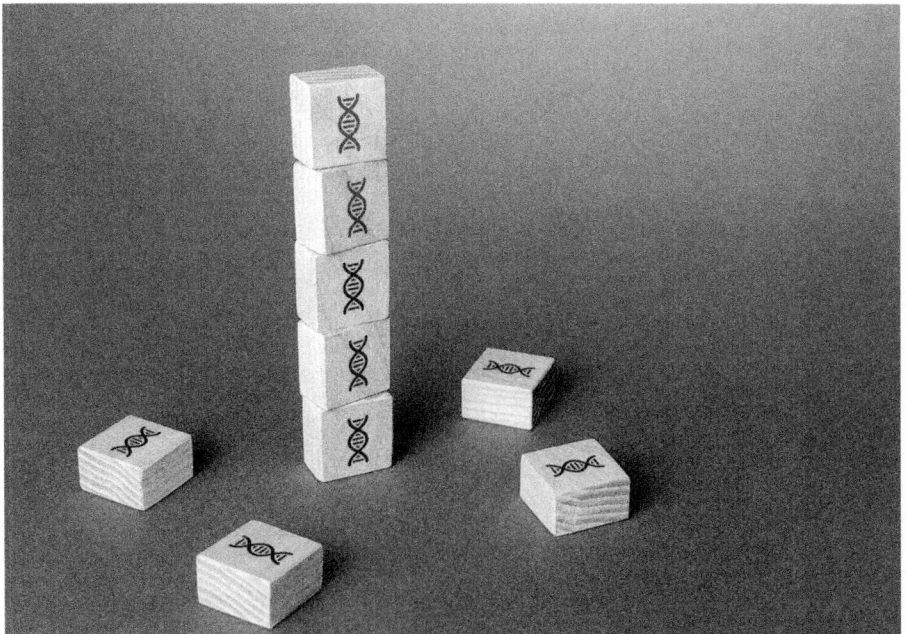

Stem cells are unspecialized cells within the human body that have the ability to divide and renew into specialized cells. It has long been known that proper nutrition increases the number of stem cells we have while junk foods and unhealthy diets can inhibit cellular restoration. However, another action that has an impact on these versatile cells is fasting.

Fasting for 24 hours greatly increases the rate of stem cell regeneration. Since stem cells play a role in our body's ability to heal itself and ward off disease by keeping internal inflammation in check, we want as many as possible and for as long as possible. Unfortunately, due to the natural aging process as well as the acceleration of the aging process by unhealthy foods, pollution, and other external factors, just like any other cells, stem cells become less potent with age. This is why, eventually, their numbers decrease and, with time, each generation of stem cells becomes less effective.

Calorie restriction was the "old" way that doctors could instruct patients to promote stem cell regeneration, but now we know fasting does it better. In fact, fasting switches the body's source of fuel from glycose to fatty acids and this particular shift seems to be the trigger that causes more active stem cells that vibrantly regenerate. Fasting to switch the stem cell regenerative switch promotes the production of white blood cells to fight infection and, according to Valter Longo, Professor of Gerontology and the Biological Sciences at the University of California, fasting for just three days can overhaul your entire immune system!

Growth Hormone (HGH)

Growth hormone is present in children as a necessary component to help them properly develop. As we get older, growth hormone is needed for strong muscles, healthy brain function, healthy cholesterol levels, bone density, and proper fat distribution. It helps the body heal, keeps metabolism high, and promotes glowing, healthy skin. Unfortunately, HGH also begins to decline around 30 years of age.

Fasting is an effective way to increase growth hormone, regardless of age. In fact, studies consistently find that 24 hours already increases growth hormone levels, but fasting for two days can result in a five-fold increase in HGH. A five-day fast results in a 300% increase and five days of fasting over 1,250%.[29] These results led to the creation of the book, *Eat Stop Eat* by bodybuilder Brad Pilon and sparked the "Lean Gains" training method by bodybuilder Martin Berkhan.

Elevated levels of HGH promote thermogenesis while maintaining muscle mass. Thermogenesis is heat production, which helps your body burn stubborn fat. When the pituitary gland secretes HGH, it quickly travels to the liver where it is converted into other types of growth factors including Insulin-Like Growth Factor 1 (IGF1) which promotes lean body mass and bone density, among other things. At the same time, glucose production rises in the liver, which creates the need for another source of energy: fat. Therefore, the entire process of HGH production and secretion helps the body mobilize and oxidize fats, which accounts for the increase in fat burning.

29   Kerndt PR, Naughton JL, Driscoll CE, Loxterkamp DA. Fasting: the history, pathophysiology and complications. West J Med. 1982 Nov;137(5):379-99. PMID: 6758355; PMCID: PMC1274154.

Building Muscle and Improved Fitness Performance

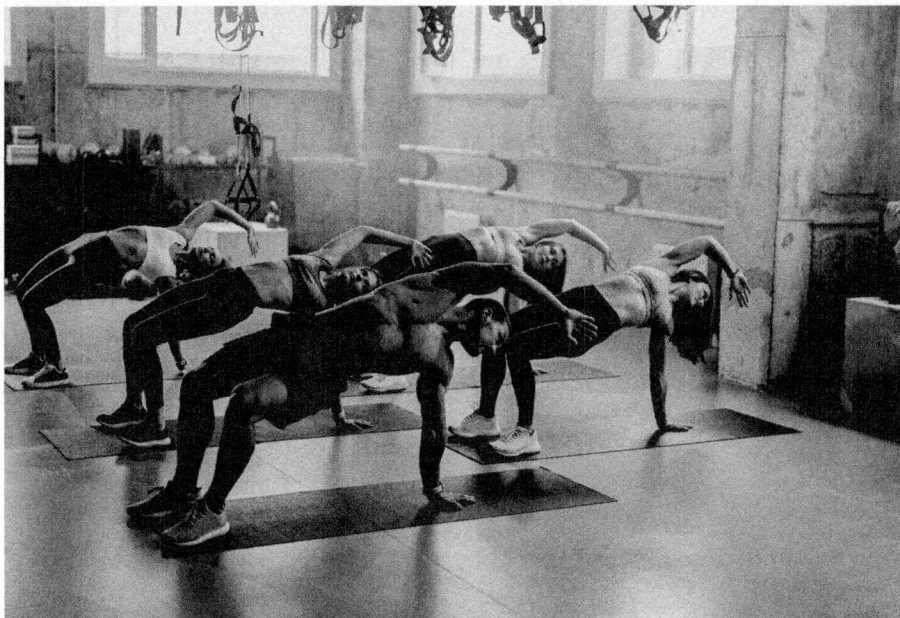

Building muscle and improved fitness performance are natural side effects of fasting. It does seem counterintuitive, thanks to misguided nutrition advice from governments and other so-called experts that have promoted the idea that we constantly need to feed the body for improved fitness. It turns out that couldn't be further from the truth. As stated earlier, our bodies thrive on fasting, as they go into survival mode and a number of functions kick in. This results in an increase in our body's ability to thrive and adapt. Therefore, we can take advantage of these natural instincts through fasting.

Furthermore, we already know from previous chapters that fasting actually burns fat and does not lead to fat storage as once thought. But as we have seen, fasting stimulates an increase in growth hormone which is necessary for building muscle. In addition, fasting forces the body to utilize energy systems more efficiently, leading to a decrease in fat stores that can slow us down. It also activates the sympathetic nervous system, which slows digestion, increases heart rate, and once again, means a breakdown of fat for energy.

To continue, the 16:8 fasting method is a popular way to quickly get in shape. If one fasts from evening or bedtime until late the following morning, the morning workout can be used to burn more fat by exercising on an empty stomach. For those who wish to build muscle, a high-quality protein powder should be consumed before strength training and followed by a high protein, low carb meal post-workout.

Each type of fasting comes with its own idiosyncrasies and each person will respond differently to fasting and training. For example, strength training might be put on hold during an extended water or dry fast. Alternate-day fasting might allow some people to continue their workout as normal, but fasting days may need to be modified (by consuming 500 – 600 calories per day). Your current level of health, as well as your goals, will define what type of exercise, if any, you can do while fasting.

No matter what type you do, try fasting without exercise before doing so with exercise in order to see how your body responds, and then, you can take it from there. Some people may have health issues that could cause fatigue during fasting to allow the body to heal. But, once complete, most fasters have far more energy for training and the body responds much better to exercise and training. Listen to your body during your fast and you will find your rhythm.

Creating Healthier Habits

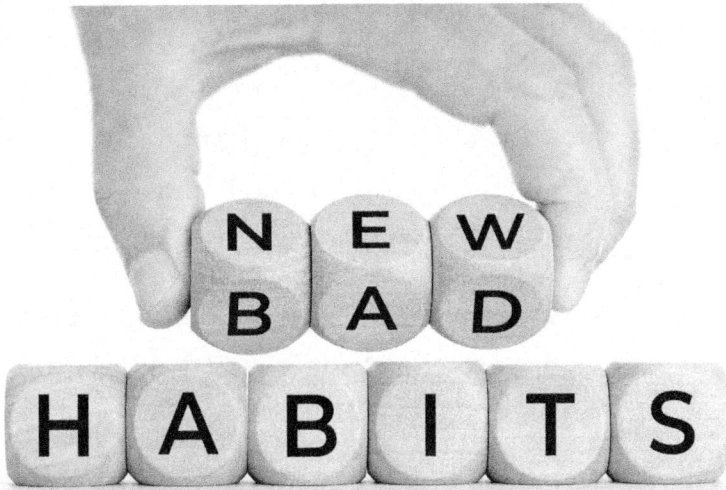

Creating healthier habits is a common side effect of fasting as it promotes the state of ketosis. One reason low-carb diets are so popular is that they are the best way to lose fat and preserve muscle. However, in addition to this, being in the state of ketosis actually suppresses hunger, so keeping your body in ketosis can help curb appetite while abstaining from carbohydrates can help curb cravings. This is a powerful combination that can help you begin to create healthier habits that will last. But there are even more ways that fasting helps with behavior control.

To start with, ghrelin is a hormone that stimulates appetite, promotes fat storage, and slows metabolism. It is secreted just before meals, but abstaining from eating disrupts the cycle and thus, the hormone. The natural assumption is that a steady intake of food will suppress ghrelin levels, but that is not the case.

It turns out that the hormone peaks at normal times associated with the mid-day meal and evening meal, however, it is lower in the morning with the lowest point being at 9 am. Interestingly, after the other mealtimes when ghrelin recedes, it does so whether you eat or not. (Natalucci G et al., European J Endo 152; 845-850) For those who ride out the waves of hunger, ghrelin tends to decrease, therefore hunger subsides making it easier to control your appetite.

Furthermore, dopamine and serotonin are both hormones associated with feelings of wellbeing. Fasting increases levels of both of these hormones, which may explain why many people have improved moods and mental attitudes while fasting. Keep in mind this may not be true for those who are new to fasting. It takes time for the body to cut through cravings and have "normal" physical responses to fasting. However, the effect fasting has on hormonal activities and other functions can help compensate while the body is learning or adjusting to fasting.

Because of the physical changes, including the hormones ghrelin, dopamine, and serotonin, appetite becomes more in control as your mood and sense of wellbeing improve. Taken together, this is a powerful combination that can help restore willpower, making it easier to install the healthy habits that will help you reach your goals.

Spiritual Benefits

Spiritual benefits are very much associated with fasting. Everything we have learned so far is that fasting has a highly positive effect on all areas of the body. This includes lowering the risk for many types of disease, improving mental health, having more discipline, and even having a natural hormonal balance. But fasting has a profound effect on our spiritual health as well.

Digestion is a process that involves a lot of internal energy such as the churning of the stomach, muscle contractions in the intestinal tract, and the release and use of many digestive enzymes throughout the entire alimentary canal. Fasting puts a stop to these processes as digestion is allowed to rest. The quiet and calm of the digestive process can translate into more energy for the brain without any excess mental signals that may come with digestion. This could account for the improved concentration skills during fasting.

Furthermore, fasting increases the production of norepinephrine and adrenaline, hormones that increase mental alertness and clarity. At the same time, dopamine is increased, thus balancing alertness with wellbeing. This may also explain why fasting is used to increase spirituality or to improve communication with higher powers.

However, there are even more reasons why fasting is associated with religion and spirituality. Many who fast simply feel more in tune with the world around them, both visible and invisible. Not eating leaves more time for meditation or prayer while improving discipline, which is also associated with becoming closer to a higher power. And lastly, fasting promotes cleansing and internal healing of all organs, including the brain, which may result in a more peaceful state of mind.

Reduced Inflammation

Reduced inflammation is a very desirable side effect of all forms of fasting. While inflammation may be a necessary part of the immune system, internal, chronic inflammation is linked to numerous diseases such as cancer and heart disease. While a healthy diet can contribute to lowered inflammation, fasting can expedite reducing inflammation even more. Fortunately, studies consistently show that 24 hours of fasting greatly reduces inflammation and it lowers oxidative stress as well, while other studies show this may take place in as little time as 12 hours.

According to Mount Sinai in New York and published in the journal, *Cell*, highly inflammatory immune cells called monocytes are the cause of internal tissue damage and are linked to chronic diseases.[30] Even worse, modern-day eating habits of foods that are highly processed and high in refined carbohydrates increase the amount we have in our blood. However, fasting seems to reduce the number of these cells and can even put them into a dormant state so they are not as harmful.

In addition to a smaller number of less active monocytes, fasting also increases the amounts of ketones in the blood. Previously, it was mentioned that ketones derived from fat become a source of fuel for the body and brain when no carbohydrates are consumed. Ketones are a superior source of energy for the brain and help burn fat as fuel, which has an effect on fat to muscle ratio. Along with these amazing benefits, ketones also help lower inflammation by inhibiting the activity of cells such as NF-kB and NLRP3, thus reducing internal inflammation.

---

30 Jordan, S., & Tung, N. (2019). Dietary Intake Regulates the Circulating Inflammatory Monocyte Pool. https://www.cell.com/cell/fulltext/S0092-8674(19)30850-5#articleInformation.

Healing Chronic Pain

Healing chronic pain and other issues is a motivator for many who embark on fasting programs. Internal inflammation can cause pain, especially in the joint pain that accompanies arthritis or abdominal pain in those who suffer from irritable bowel syndrome (IBS). Pain is often the result of inflammation, and over-the-counter pain medications, like ibuprofen, are used to reduce it. But as we saw above, fasting helps reduce chronic inflammation and thus reduces pain as well. This makes fasting a less invasive and less expensive way of dealing with pain. Of course, to keep pain at bay, helping your body heal with the right foods on non-fasting days is imperative.

A few years ago, I was lucky enough to heal a chronic shoulder pain that lasted for 2 years. Some days it was completely debilitating, but after a 10-day water fast, the pain went away completely and permanently. I also haven't had a single flare-up of eczema since. But enough about me!

Decrease in Metabolic Diseases

A decrease in metabolic diseases is another leading motivation for those who fast. Metabolic diseases cover a wide range of health issues that may be due to genetics, lifestyle or environment. Here, I am specifically referring to the group known as chronic, metabolic diseases, which are often self-inflicted yet afflict the majority of the world population who follow a standard or typical modern diet and a sedentary lifestyle.

These diseases include obesity, diabetes, liver and cardiovascular disease, and all of these can be addressed through fasting. Fasting helps lower calorie intake and triggers hormonal changes that affect metabolism and even hormones associated with hunger. Therefore, planned and regular fasting protocols can help improve weight. As fasting helps to improve blood sugar levels, the risk of diabetes can lessen and may be brought under control. By lowering internal inflammation and oxidative stress, as mentioned earlier, you will also lower the risk for cardiovascular and liver diseases. It is also worth mentioning that when the body undergoes autophagy, which lessens toxins and reduces inflammation, all the organs, including your liver, have more energy that can be used for natural healing processes and cell regeneration.

Improved Digestion

Better digestion is a side effect of fasting for a number of reasons. Autophagy, the process of detoxification discussed above, extends into the digestive tract where it repairs and regenerates the gut lining. This leads to an improved microbiome, the home of our healthy flora and microbes that not only aid digestion, but play a role in many other areas, including healthy hormonal balance. Just like any other area of the body, when allowed to rest, the microbiome can naturally reset and balance for improved digestion.

Just 24 hours of fasting can greatly increase digestive enzyme activity throughout the entire digestive system. Our survival instincts have always relied on feast and famine, with famine or lack of food being the time digestion can rest and the body clears waste, instead. But in today's world of consuming meals and then heavy beverages and snacks in between meals, the digestive system never has time to rest. This creates a situation where the digestive cycle never has time to work and then rest, and food is never completely digested. But fasting can give your digestion the much-needed downtime it needs to reset itself to normal levels, as your natural circadian rhythm takes over.

Balancing Hormones

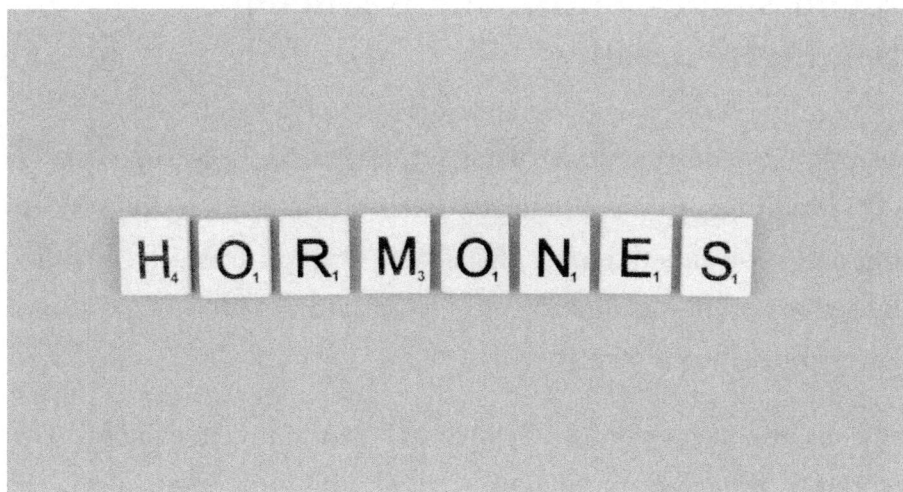

Balanced hormones is a natural side effect of fasting. As I keep mentioning throughout this book, fasting improves insulin levels as well as levels of many other hormones, such as dopamine and epinephrine. What many people don't realize is that hormones do not work individually, but synergistically or together as one unit. All hormonal levels rely on the hormonal levels of other hormones to balance, with growth hormone being at the base.

As we have seen, fasting can greatly increase the amount of growth hormone in both men and women of any age. It helps improve levels of hunger hormones and those associated with happiness and wellbeing. In men, fasting improves communication of a hormone called gonadotropin-releasing hormone (GnRH) to the gonads resulting in increased testosterone, while in women fasting affects the hormones and precursors that are linked to healthy estrogen levels. *(Note how fasting affects sex hormone levels in women greatly depends upon medications, such as birth control as well as the level of health.)*

Blood Sugar Control and Reducing Insulin Resistance

Blood sugar control and reducing insulin resistance are two benefits of fasting that are directly linked to each other. When food is continuously consumed, especially carbohydrates, carbs are converted into glucose and insulin moves glucose into the blood, and thus it lowers blood sugar levels.

A constant barrage of carbohydrates can cause the pancreas to work overtime and manufacture insulin at a high rate, causing the body to stop responding to it. The pancreas then works even harder by putting out more insulin as blood sugar rises, therefore, causing even more resistance. Because of this, a cycle that can lead to diabetes is born. If this continues for too long, the pancreas eventually gets to a point when it can no longer make insulin, which can become very dangerous.

Fasting naturally lessens blood sugar while regular fasting has an overall positive effect on how the body manages blood sugar and insulin. While the mechanisms are not completely understood, many people use intermittent fasting to improve blood sugar levels, so they feel better all day. As I mentioned previously, fasting helps balance hormones and allows the body to reset itself. Moreover, since insulin is a hormone, it may be affected in a positive way as we also abstain from all food, and thus, incoming blood sugar.

Improved Heart Health

Fasting affects a number of physiological factors that play a role in cardiovascular health, including lower blood pressure. This effect is so profound that a study published in the Journal of the American Heart Association stated participants on medications for blood pressure were able to stop medications with fasting. (Grundler et al., 2020)

Another improvement that takes place during fasting is that blood triglycerides, or fats, are lowered. This is because during fasting the body uses fat to burn energy instead of glucose. Regular fasting leads to consistently lower blood triglycerides, which also helps lower cholesterol levels and blood sugar. This is a win-win benefit for your entire body!

Boost Brain Function and Prevent Neurodegenerative Disorders

Fasting is the ideal way to boost cognitive function and prevent neurodegenerative diseases. We already mentioned that, while fasting, your body must use fats for energy instead of glucose. These fats are turned into ketones, which are a more efficient form of energy for the brain. This leads to improved brain function together with greater clarity and focus.

Because fasting helps reduce the risk of and can help heal metabolic diseases, the risk of neurological disease is also lowered as metabolic diseases can affect brain health. In addition, fasting induces an altered or heightened metabolic state in which the body can heal and regenerate from head to toe. This action improves brain plasticity and resilience while optimizing neuron bioenergetics, and together these actions lead to protection from brain diseases, including tumors.[31]

Aid in Cancer Prevention and Increase the Effectiveness of Chemotherapy

Fasting increases the number of stem cells we have available, which are cells that assist in healing and regeneration. These same stem cells also regenerate the immune system and increase the production of tumor-killing cells. When used correctly, fasting also helps you lose weight, which can reduce the risk of obesity or lower one's weight out of the range considered obese. And since many cancers have obesity as a risk fact, this is a twofold benefit of fasting. But it gets better.

Fasting helps cancer patients tolerate chemotherapy better while making treatment more effective. This is because fasting and chemotherapy combined caused the body to produce higher amounts of lymphocytes and common lymphoid progenitor cells, both of which create white blood cells that are known to kill tumors. In the same study, fasting helped protect normal, healthy cells while che-

---

31   Phillips MCL. Fasting as a Therapy in Neurological Disease. Nutrients. 2019;11(10):2501. Published 2019 Oct 17. doi:10.3390/nu11102501

motherapy still killed cancer cells. When combined with the benefit of increased stem cell production, it is clear that fasting can have profound benefits in preventing cancer as well as healing.

Detoxification

Cellular detoxification is the natural process that is called autophagy. When the body is not using resources to digest and process food, it can turn the energy toward this natural process. We see this in not only autophagy, but also when the body switches to using ketones for energy instead of glucose. The process becomes even more intense when dry fasting as the body uses metabolic water and toxins from fats for energy, thus destroying the toxins in the process. This makes fasting a highly effective form of natural detoxification without the fuss of costly herbs and supplements.

Sexual Health and Performance

For men, fasting increases testosterone levels without the side effects of medications or synthetic hormones. Women who fast see an overall improvement in hormonal balance while both genders enjoy the benefit of increased growth hormone. When combined, these physiological changes can improve libido and sexual health.

At the same time, fasting improves mental outlook as the hormones dopamine and serotonin are increased, leading to more self-confidence, especially when combined with any weight loss that occurs. Increased energy, confidence, and a happier mood all lead to improved sexual health and performance that can benefit both partners without the need for medications, while overall health improves. This can lead to a healthy cycle of improved physical health and relationships.

Side Effects or the Healing Crisis

It is important to note that in all forms of fasting, the extent or severity of the side effects depends upon your level of health when you begin the fast and the preparation you put into the fast. If you do not prepare your body for a fast, you will experience more side effects than benefits. This does not mean you don't receive benefits; it only means you won't feel as good during the fast.

To conclude, I highly recommend that you get ready for a fast by physically preparing your body with the right foods leading up to the fast as well as getting mentally prepared by planning your schedule. Planning will help you in all areas such as what days you will fast, having the proper foods on hand to break the fast, what you will do to occupy your time during the fast, and ideas that will help you overcome obstacles.

How to Get Started and Then Break Your Fast

Preparing for Your Fast

Consult with your doctor. This goes for any fast or any practice that I have listed in this book. This is especially true for anyone with a medical condition or taking medications, even if the medication is birth control. Never fast while on medications without consulting your doctor and never stop taking your medications without the okay from your doctor, first.

Preparing your life circumstances might also be helpful for fasting. If you have a family and are usually the "designated" meal planner, then plan something ahead of time that is easy for them to prepare or cook. If your children rely on you and are old enough, this is a great time to begin teaching them to be self-sufficient (this pertains to partners, as well).

Plan a schedule of the days you will eat normally and the days you will fast. If you will do intermittent fasting (IF), write out a weekly schedule. If you will do an extended water fast, plan out the days you will prepare your body and the meals leading up to your fast as well as the food you will use to come out of your fast. Statistically, people who plan out their days like this are far more successful with sticking to their health goals.

Get Ready

I am certain one reason why fasting has a bad reputation with some people is that they go about it wrong. Fasting is an extreme and very effective form of natural detoxification and from all the science we have seen, it is also an instinctively healthy and beneficial practice. It helps the body reset many functions that are connected to the circadian rhythm and in most cases leaves a person in better health than when they began. So, what happened?

The problem is that many people do not properly prepare their bodies for fasting. In natural health, we know that your body reacts negatively in proportion to the number of toxins and waste that are built up in the system. This means that the more excess waste you have in your body, the more difficult it is for your body to get rid of it. It takes a lot of internal energy to detoxify and remove internal waste, and if you are not strong enough or hydrated enough, your body simply does not have the energy to do the work.

But if you ease into a fast with proper "training," you will get the most benefits with the least problems or side effects. First, if you want to feel great during your fast, it is best to start in ketosis, however, it is not necessary. When you begin fasting, your body will naturally move into ketosis as it begins to utilize ketones from fat for energy instead of glucose from carbohydrates.

Putting your body into ketosis is a smoother route to help your body transition without the shock of going into ketosis while abstaining from food at the same time, which is why some experts recommend it. The following steps can help you get there.

- **Stop eating junk foods**, fast foods, and highly processed foods as much as possible. This includes most restaurant foods, desserts, and sugary snacks. If you have a habit of eating these foods, keep in mind that abstaining from them gets easier even after the first day, especially if you avoid carbs.
- **Begin reducing carbohydrates** as much as possible. This first step may feel confusing at first because it is best to begin learning how many carbs are in all the foods you eat. However, this becomes a habit a lot quicker than most people realize as many of us do not vary our meals much. In many cases, people consume the same breakfasts, snacks, and lunches as every other day, especially during a workweek. If you don't, then try using similar meals to learn the carbs of the foods you eat.
- **Pay attention to proteins** and try to consume a small amount of protein and healthy fat with each meal or snack. As you transition away from carbs, begin to keep track of your carbohydrate, protein, and fat intake to help your body transition into ketosis. The goal is to consume 70% of your calories from healthy fats (much easier than it sounds since fats have a lot of calories), 25% of your calories from healthy proteins, and 5% from carbohydrates.

- **Learn macronutrient rations.** The above ratio of 70% fat / 25% protein / 5% carbs is considered a Standard Keto Diet (SKD). However, there are easier versions if it suits you, such as the Targeted Keto Diet (TKD) comprising 65-70% fat / 20% protein / 10-15% carbs or the High Protein Keto Diet (HPKD) for very active people, which is 60-65% fat / 30% protein / 5-10% carbs. While practicing with macronutrient ratios may feel intimidating or complicated at first, most people find it much easier after just two or three days. It is okay to play around with the numbers to find your "sweet spot."

(If you are in perimenopause or menopause, many experts now recommend prioritizing protein, consuming a lower percentage of fat, and still restricting carbohydrates.)

- **Tighten your diet for at least 2-3 weeks** to help your body go into ketosis. This is not necessary; however, it will really help you get the most from your fast and your efforts. Fasting is much easier when your body is in ketosis, and feeling great allows you to focus on other things in your life instead of trying to deal with side effects.

- **Consume coconut oil** as part of your diet. Coconut oil contains MCTs or medium-chain fatty acids that are easily utilized by the liver. This helps your body to more easily adjust to using ketones for energy while at the same time increasing thermogenesis, or the heat effect, which can help you burn an extra 120 or more calories a day.

- **Exercise at least 3-5 days** each week while putting your body into ketosis. When you exercise, your body burns glycogen, including any that may be stored, forcing your body to then rely on ketones for fuel. When combined with the above macronutrient ratios in your diet, you should go into ketosis more easily. Also note that if the low-carb diet is new to you, your energy levels may be low, so physical activity should also be reduced. You can still exercise but stick to walking, stretching, yoga, and other forms of healthy and low-key activities.

- **Drink plenty of fresh spring water.** Also begin to reduce your intake of caffeinated beverages and alcohol, which will help reduce side effects during your fast.

If you are anxious to get started, then do the above for at least 4-7 days before beginning your fast. This will still help you transition, get your body ready, and mentally prepare yourself for your fast before you begin. And always keep in mind that preparation will help you succeed more easily.

Some people may not be interested in putting the body into ketosis before they fast, and that's okay. If this sounds like you, then follow these steps to help you prepare for your fast.

- **Stop eating junk foods** and highly processed foods like frozen meals, pastries, candies, and other foods that are not close to their natural form. The more junk food you consume close to your fast, the worse you will feel during your fast.
- **Greatly reduce refined carbohydrates** like bread, pasta, and any other foods that use white or bleached flour. Again, the more you eat these close to your fast, the worse you will feel.
- **Consume high-quality proteins** and healthy fats. Include foods like beef, poultry, fish, avocadoes, soaked nuts, peas, seeds, lentils, and beans. Only consume one serving of protein at a meal with-

out overeating. Consuming plenty of protein will help you feel stronger when you do fast.

- **Add raw and cooked vegetables** to your daily meal, as well as one or two servings of raw fruit, such as berries. This will aid your digestion by helping it clear a bit, making your fast more productive and more comfortable.
- **If you don't exercise**, try adding daily stretching, walking, or yoga to stimulate blood flow and movement in your lymphatic system. This will help you remove more waste during your fast. Rebounding is another great way to get the lymphatic system going.
- **Drink plenty of fresh spring water.** Also begin to reduce your intake of caffeinated beverages and alcohol, which will help reduce side effects during your fast.

Ease into All Fasting

Even after you have "trained" your body to fast, you should still ease into it. This is true for both water and dry fasts as well as intermittent fasting. The difference lies in how you ease into the fast you are going to do. As mentioned, no matter which type of fast you decide to follow, do your best to physically prepare your body by following the above guidelines to either go into ketosis or to get stronger. Then try the following.

Intermittent Fasting: Plan the hours you will fast and healthy meals for when you eat. If your goal of IF utilizes a longer fasting window like 16:8, go as long as you can the first time you abstain from eating for 16 hours. Remember that IF allows water, black coffee, and tea during fasting periods, so do your best while remaining within these guidelines. If 16:8 is too long then try shorter fasting periods like 14:10 until you reach your goal.

Alternate Day Fasting: These are the fasts including OMAD or 5:3 where you will fast for an entire 24 hours. During this fast, you are also allowed water, black coffee, and tea. Do your best to fast the entire 24 hours, but if you cannot, use the modified methods of eating 500 calories in two or three small meals during your fasting days. Drinking a small cup of bone broth is another way to get over the difficult times. Again, planning your meals and shopping ahead of time will greatly increase your chance of success.

Water Fasting: If your goal is to water fast for 24 hours or longer, then practice with the above method of Alternate Day Fasting and do your best to go an entire 24 hours. If you don't succeed, you can always try again. Always listen to your body and stop if you are not feeling well!

Be sure to have activities planned to take your mind off of eating. Some activities to include are taking a bath, meditating, taking a walk, reading, or cleaning your home. Now is a great time to work on a side business or begin a new hobby. Many people learn to enjoy their fasting days when they realize how many other things they can get done while not preoccupied with food or planning meals.

You will also learn the difference between "true hunger" and just wanting to eat or snack out of habit or boredom.

Dry Fasting: Only try this if you are very experienced with different fasting methods and have done extended water fasts.

Begin incorporating small time slots of dry fasting as part of your IF plan. You can also include some dry fasting days during a longer water fast. Remember you are in charge and if you truly need to drink water you can and you should. But do all things with caution, even drinking water after a short period of dry fasting because you have to "wake up" your digestive tract after its resting period.

If you need help, plan on having a support system, such as a health practitioner, friends, or an online or local fasting group. A support system can help you through the tough times and be a great source of information if you are unsure and have questions about your experience. And above all else, be safe, pay attention to your body. Remember that you have control over your health and easing into new health practices is far easier than harming yourself.

How to Break your Fast

Breaking your fast is almost more important than preparing for it. While fasting, your digestion has switched from breaking down food to autophagy (along with other physiological changes). Eating a large meal of the wrong foods can cause stomach upset, bloating, cramps, and other symptoms of digestive distress and possibly sabotage your health goals. Instead, ease back into eating with the following guidelines.

- Begin with sips of water if you have been dry fasting. Allow your body time to absorb the water by slowly sipping for the first hour or so. The longer you dry fast, the longer you should take to allow your body to come out of it. Take your time and pay attention to your stomach and digestive system to know how quickly you can move to food.

- For all types of fasting, begin eating with a small amount of raw, organic fruit. Apples are a great choice thanks to their natural fiber and enzymes. It is best to avoid fruit that is very high in sugar, such as bananas.

- Sipping broth or consuming a small meal of steamed vegetables is another option to begin breaking your fast.

- Chew all food thoroughly and slowly to allow your body time to create and excrete digestive enzymes. Also, take your time eating to allow the muscles of your digestive tract to fully work again. Remember they play an active role in digestion as the stomach contracts and churns to aid digestion and the intestinal tract uses peristalsis, or wave-like motions to move food through.

- After a few hours, incorporate a small meal of cooked vegetables and protein. Be sure to continue sipping water throughout the day, as well.

- If you have been using an IF plan, then your fast will be broken with similar foods each day. Choose your meals wisely and pay attention to how you feel after each meal. This will help you get a sense of what your body can tolerate or not.

- After fasting, strive to only eat foods that are within the guidelines of your meal plan and avoid junk foods and highly processed foods. This is a great time to practice discipline and get to know your body.

The above are traditional guidelines for breaking a fast and are commonly used for most diets that will be used after the fast. Ultimately, the goal is to slowly awaken the digestive system and then ease back into a healthy diet plan. With that being said, I do things a bit differently, as my normal diet plan is a keto/carnivore diet.

If you're on a keto, carnivore, or low-carb diet, then you would want to follow Dr. Mindy's recommendations for breaking your fast, which would look more like this:

How to Break a Fast
Greater than 24 hours
4-Step Process

1   BONE BROTH
Contains glycine that repairs
the inner lining of the gut.

2   PROBIOTIC FOOD
Replenishes the gut with good bacteria
(sauerkraut, kombucha, yogurt, kimchi)

3   STEAMED VEGGIES
Provides fiber to the good bacteria

4   PROTEIN
Ready now for animal or plant protein

Dr Mindy Pelz

CHAPTER 6

Troubleshooting

I ADDED THIS SECTION FOR THOSE WHO MIGHT HAVE QUESTIONS about the fasting process and need answers. Very often while fasting, many people share problems like headaches, nausea, or foggy mind. Why these side effects happen is very individual because they may happen for different reasons; for example, some people may experience headaches as withdrawal from caffeine, while others experience headaches due to dehydration or an electrolyte imbalance. I will add below some common symptoms or side effects and offer several ways to deal with them, so you can try each and see what works for you. But first I will address exercise and fasting to provide some insight on how to either incorporate it or continue it, depending upon your fasting plan.

Exercise while Fasting

Exercise during a fast works for some while others need to rest during this time. It depends on your level of health and exercise history as well as what type of fast you are doing and why you are doing it.

Generally speaking, modified fasts in which you consume $500 - 600$ calories a day are the type of fasts in which you can continue exercising and even doing the same exercises that you have already been doing. However, if you have never exercised and want to incorporate some form of it, begin very slowly and on the non-fasting days. Allow your body time to adjust and become stronger before you take on any intense strength training or endurance cardio training.

Extended water and dry fasting are times when your body moves energy into detoxification, healing, and repair. Incorporating exercise during this time can take the energy away from these processes, which works against the goals of the diet. At the same time, your muscles may not have the energy for intense exercise of any kind.

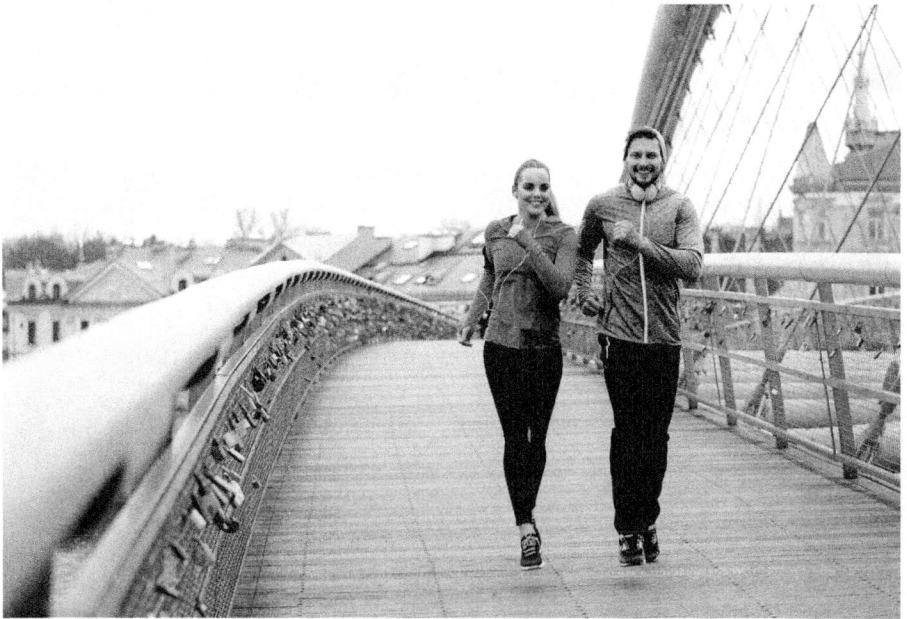

During these more intense phases of fasting, modify your workouts so that they are low-level with less weight and/or less intensity. Incorporate more workouts that are centered around stretching and yoga, which can also be forms of meditation. Moderate-paced walking can also be used and can help promote blood flow as well as lymphatic flow, both of which will help your body clear the waste and toxins that it may be dislodging. If you don't exercise, you can still incorporate these into a semi-daily routine to enhance the benefits of fasting.

For certain fasts like the OMAD or the ADF programs, strength training may be incorporated. As mentioned previously, some athletes including runners and bodybuilders find that this type of fasting enhances their strength training and allows them to get stronger. If you decide to begin strength training after fasting, employ the help of a professional trainer and nutritionist to guide you.

Troubleshooting

The following are some typical fasting and detoxification side effects and how to deal with them.

Dizziness is common as toxins are dislodged from all areas of your body, including the brain. But dizziness may also be an indication of an electrolyte imbalance or dehydration. If you experience dizziness, check your activity level to be sure you're not overdoing it. Also, sip water with lemon with a pinch of salt. If you need a full-on electrolyte drink, mix the following:

- 4 ounces of spring water (or as much as you require)
- ¼ tsp Himalayan pink salt
- 1/8 cup freshly squeezed lemon juice
- 1 cup unsweetened coconut water (for potassium)
- 1 tsp raw honey or pure maple syrup (also potassium)

Some people swear by the **Snake Juice** combination for fasting:

- 2 liters of water
- 2g (½ tsp) of Himalayan pink salt
- 5g (1 tsp) of salt-free potassium chloride
- 2g (½ tsp) of food-grade Epsom salt

Dizziness may also be a sign that your body is switching from glucose to ketones for fuel. This will pass and the drinks should help.

During dry fasts, I will put pink Himalayan salt crystals under my tongue as needed.

Headaches are very common, especially for those who normally drink caffeine. Low blood sugar, dehydration, and caffeine or sugar withdrawal can all be triggers for headaches. Make sure you are hydrated and if necessary, try the electrolyte drink above. Also, rest as much as possible, and keep a cool or warm moist cloth on your head, whichever works for you. Headaches from fasting are usually very temporary and stop happening with regular fasting practice.

Low Blood Sugar is somewhat common and is more often due to the body switching from using glucose as fuel to ketones instead. While it is still a form of low blood sugar, this is the goal, and the body needs time to adapt to using ketones. This state is not a danger to health unless you have rare or existing conditions. Most fasters try to work through this with electrolyte drinks, or bone broth to provide protein for energy or consume more protein during normal eating days.

Irregular Heartbeat may take place due to electrolyte imbalances. Try the drinks above and be sure to rest. Anyone with a medical condition should talk to his/her medical provider about the right diet during non-fasting periods or do a modified form of fasting and include protein in the 500 – 600 fasting day calories. Potassium supplements may work for some, but usually, a doctor will prescribe this. Drinking an electrolyte drink can also provide the potassium necessary during fasting.

Hunger is an issue for most during fasting. Drinking water and tea is the best way to curb the feeling of an empty stomach. Also, keep in mind that your circadian rhythm will cause a rise in hunger during midday and early evening, which are considered the normal times to eat a meal. When you don't eat, the hunger feeling actually subsides. Also use patience, knowing that your hunger hormones such as ghrelin are being reset.

Sleep Issues occur in some people who fast and may be due to a number of reasons. First, remember the process of autophagy in which the body destroys and removes spent or damaged cells. This may also take place in the brain and some experts theorize this process can cause sleep disturbances. Also, the sleep cycle is part of the circadian rhythm and so interrelated with the hunger pattern. A temporary disturbance in hunger may trigger more brain energy and make it difficult to sleep. The best remedy may be a hot bath with Epsom salt and lavender oil to help relax your body and mind. Moreover, be sure you are drinking enough water if you are not dry fasting. Incorporate mindfulness practices throughout the day to help reduce anxiety, such as relaxation techniques and meditation.

Becoming Hangry is a problem for some. This may be due to de-hydration and of course, being hungry. Keep in mind that hunger waves come and go, so try to meditate or breathe through them. Drink water if necessary to keep your stomach full, or drink green tea to curb your appetite. Drink high-quality vegetables or bone broth if the lack of nutrients is really bothering you. Brush your teeth to abate hunger and keep yourself busy with hobbies or other activities to keep your mind off of food. Sometimes it takes practice, but if you can get your mind to a healthy state where you are enjoying the healing process, you might find that being "hangry" was a mental state of a past, unhealthier version of you.

Bathroom Issues like constipation and/or diarrhea affect some who fast. If you are constipated, keep in mind that you are not eating and so this may be a normal state. Taking a mild herbal laxative before your fast might help clear the intestinal tract, thus reducing any full feelings in the bowels. Also, make sure you are hydrated to help avoid this problem, and if you take fiber supplements be aware you may need more water.

On one hand, some people choose to do regular or even daily enemas (also coffee enemas) while fasting and others get regular colonics. These can be utilized periodically to increase cleansing and detoxification of the liver and intestines.

On the other hand, other people experience diarrhea, which may be due to the body attempting to heal a parasitic infection or other types of microbial imbalance. Taking a fiber supplement during non-fasting days may help improve your situation as well as abstaining from coffee. Be sure to drink an electrolyte drink to avoid dehydration. If your issue is extreme, a medical test might be in order.

Feeling Cold is quite common while fasting. Body temperature usually decreases during a fast, along with blood pressure, pulse, and respiratory rate. This is further evidence of the inherent wisdom of the body to conserve energy. You might need to dress a bit warmer than usual or turn the indoor temperature up. You can also try hot baths, infrared saunas, drinking hot tea, and using hot water bottles, to stay warm.

Medications should be discussed with your medical doctor before fasting, and preferably with the doctor who prescribed the medication. In some cases, taking medication during religious fasting is considered breaking the fast, and again, should be discussed with your doctor.

Female Issues when Fasting

Unfortunately, some female issues do arise during fasting. Some may be normal and some may not, and experiencing them will depend on your health history, the current level of health, and any medications that you take or have taken in the past. Some of the following are some female issues that may arise while fasting.

Increased menstruation may take place for some women, especially younger women. This is because fasting begins the processes of autophagy and autolysis, both of which break down expired, damaged, or diseased tissues for removal. Menstruation is a woman's "normal" detoxification cycle during which the body sheds the lining of the uterus that is not used for pregnancy. During fasting, this process may become stronger as the body removes older, built-up waste, thanks to more energy being directed at these detoxification processes instead of digestion.

Lack of menstruation may take place for some women. This is not common but can happen in those who already have irregular periods or who greatly restrict their calories. Underweight women should not fast until their bodies are strong enough to do so.

Increased cortisol levels are one effect that fasting has on everyone, including healthy women.[32] Fasting is a form of stress to the body, and cortisol is one reaction to it. At the same time, some in the medical community claim that cortisol is only a result of stress, however, refined foods that are high in sugar are known to increase cortisol, as well. Since many women suffer from excess abdominal weight due to cortisol, fasting might make the situation worse, especially for those who are highly stressed or overworked. If this sounds like you, it may be best to stick with easier forms of IF or incorporate stress reduction practices to allow for safer fasting.

Thyroid hormones may drop during fasting, especially T3. T3 is a necessary hormone the body requires for energy, but while you fast, your body goes into conservation mode to save energy. This drop in hormones often resumes to healthier levels after fasting. With that being said, if you are on thyroid medications, consult with your doctor before embarking on any type of fasting.

Breast cancer patients should consider 13-hour fasting periods when using IF. In one study, 2,413 patients with early-stage breast cancer who fasted less than 13 hours showed a statistically significant in-

---

32   Mazurak, N., Günther, A., Grau, F. et al. Effects of a 48-h fast on heart rate variability and cortisol levels in healthy female subjects. Eur J Clin Nutr 67, 401–406 (2013). https://doi.org/10.1038/ejcn.2013.32

crease in a risk for recurrence compared to those who fasted longer than 13 hours. The study concluded that incorporating nightly fasting of longer than 13 hours may be a dietary strategy to reduce the risk of breast cancer recurrence in women. [33]

Overall, we each have special needs and requirements that should be paid attention to, which is why I constantly advocate consulting with your doctor before embarking on any fasting program. With that being said, fasting is an overall therapeutic tool that anyone can use to improve reproductive health, protect bones and muscles, promote the body's internal healing mechanisms, provide more energy, and control weight.

In today's world of overeating, many people find it refreshing to give digestion a rest and allow energy to flow into other areas of the body. With enhanced mental acuity, increased brain neuroplasticity (the ability to generate new learning pathways), and greater creativity, fasting is a practice worth learning and incorporating for a lifetime.

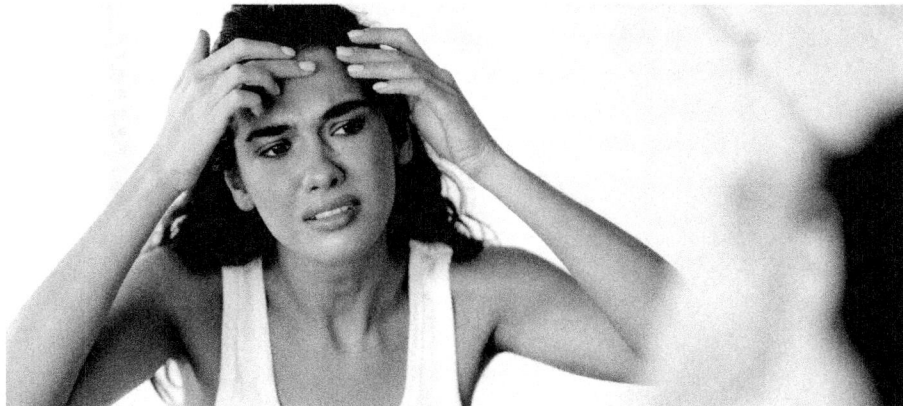

33 Marinac CR, Nelson SH, Breen CI, et al. Prolonged Nightly Fasting and Breast Cancer Prognosis. JAMA Oncol. 2016;2(8):1049-1055. doi:10.1001/jamaoncol.2016.0164

Frequently asked questions about fasting

1. **Can anyone start a fasting program?**

   Anyone can start a fasting program except for people with eating disorders, women who are pregnant or breastfeeding, and people who are under medication or have certain diseases. However, it's always recommended that you first consult with your doctor before embarking on any fasting program.

2. **Are there age restrictions for fasting?**

   It's recommended that those under 18 years of age don't follow a fasting program and that those over 70 don't follow the Fasting Mimicking Diet. However, you should speak with your doctor first.

3. **Which is the best fast for beginners?**

   Intermittent fasting programs are the safest to perform for beginners and it's suggested that you begin with short fasting periods.

4. **What is the best way to get ready for fasting?**

   Before beginning any fasting program you should consult with your doctor, especially if you're taking medications or have a medical condition. Once you have done so, decide on which days you will fast, keep track of your diet in the days leading up to the fast, and begin implementing certain changes in what you eat and drink. Stop eating junk foods, begin reducing carbohydrates, pay close attention to proteins, work on your rations, drink plenty of water, and exercise for at least 3-5 days.

5. **Which is the best fast for weight loss?**

Although most fasting programs are good for weight loss, the most popular for that purpose is Intermittent fasting 16/8. However, it will always depend on what you eat during the feeding window and how well you stick to the program.

6. **Which fast should I follow to maintain my weight?**

The best fasting program for maintaining weight would be Intermittent Fasting as you can do it regularly without any issues or big changes to your lifestyle.

7. **Which is the best fast for building muscle?**

The best fasting program for building muscle is OMAD because the body converts defective proteins as a fuel supply, instead of muscle protein. Moreover, the body releases hormones like somatropin, which preserve muscles. Intermittent Fasting 16/8 is also a very popular fasting method to get in shape fast.

8. **Can I follow a fast program if I'm vegetarian?**

The best fasting program for vegetarians is Juice fasting which consists of abstaining from solid foods and replacing meals with blended fresh fruits and vegetables, instead.

9. **Are there side effects to fasting?**

There are positive side effects to fasting such as better digestion, balanced hormones, better sexual health and performance, and more. Extended fasting can also cause fatigue, brain fog, nausea, and less commonly, hormonal disruptions. However, the side effects are highly individual as it will depend on how used you are to fasting and on your health conditions.

10. **Can fasting affect my sleep?**

Fasting may affect your sleep since the process of autophagy may also take place in the brain. The best remedy can be a hot bath with Epsom salt and lavender oil which will help relax your body and mind. Moreover, make sure you're drinking enough water (if you aren't dry fasting), and practice meditation and relaxation techniques throughout the day.

11. **Is there a fast with no calorie restriction?**

There are fasting programs with no strict calorie restrictions, such as Intermittent Fasting 16/8 or Alternate Day Fasting. However, if you want better results, you should leave unhealthy food out of your diet.

12. **Can I exercise while fasting?**

Some people can exercise during fasting and others need to rest. This will not only depend on your level of health and exercise history, but also on the type of fast you're following and your reason behind it.

13. Which is the best way to manage hunger while fasting?

Drinking water and tea is the best way to curb the feeling of hunger. Bear in mind that hunger waves come and go so you should also be patient since your hunger hormones are being reset.

14. When should I break the fast for better results?

The best moment to break a fast will depend on your particular reasons for having started a fasting program and how far you initially were from your goal. If you have doubts, you should always consult with your doctor.

15. Which is the best way to break the fast?

Breaking the fast is as important as preparing for it. You can begin eating a small amount of raw, organic fruit, such as apples. You can also sip broth or consume a small meal of steamed vegetables. Moreover, chew all your food thoroughly and slowly. After a few hours, incorporate a small meal of cooked vegetables and protein.

16. Do infusions break the fasting?

Most fasting programs allow infusions during fasting periods, such as black coffee and tea. They won't break the fasting as long as you don't add any sweeteners or dairy products.

Printed in Great Britain
by Amazon